Discovering the True You with Ayurveda

macropate

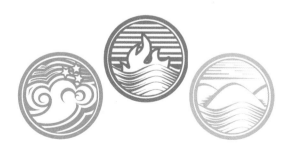

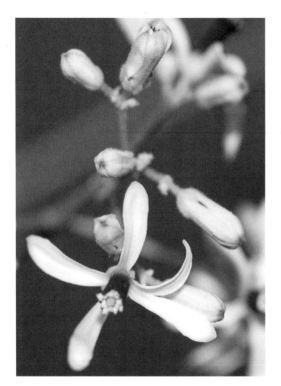
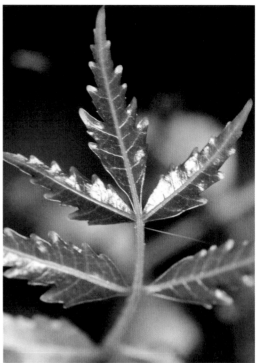
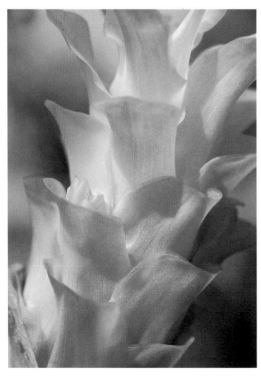
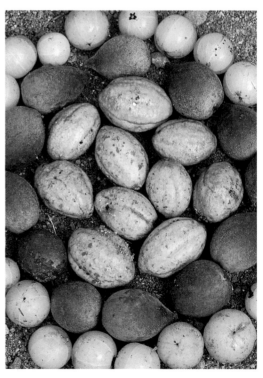

Discovering the True You with Ayurveda

How to Nourish, Rejuvenate, and Transform Your Life

SEBASTIAN POLE

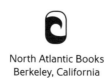

North Atlantic Books
Berkeley, California

Published by
North Atlantic Books
P.O. Box 12327
Berkeley, California 94712

Text © Sebastian Pole
Photographs © Sebastian Pole
Except: p.5, p.94 (top right, bottom left), p.174, p. 194
© Ben Heron
Design and Layout © Quadrille Publishing Ltd

Editorial Director Anne Furniss
Creative Director Helen Lewis
Project Editor Pauline Savage
Editorial Assistant Louise McKeever
Designer Nicola Davidson
Illustrator Joy FitzSimmons
Additional Elements The Space
Production Director Vincent Smith, Leonie Kellman
Printed in China

MEDICAL DISCLAIMER: The following information is intended for general information purposes only. Individuals should always see their health care provider before administering any suggestions made in this book. Any application of the material set forth in the following pages is at the reader's discretion and is his or her sole responsibility.

Discovering the True You with Ayurveda: How to Nourish, Rejuvenate, and Transform Your Life is sponsored by the Society for the Study of Native Arts and Sciences, a nonprofit educational corporation whose goals are to develop an educational and cross-cultural perspective linking various scientific, social, and artistic fields; to nurture a holistic view of arts, sciences, humanities, and healing; and to publish and distribute literature on the relationship of mind, body, and nature.

North Atlantic Books' publications are available through most bookstores. For further information, visit our website at www.northatlanticbooks.com or call 800-733-3000.

Library of Congress Cataloging-in-Publication Data

Pole, Sebastian.
  Discovering the True You with Ayurveda : How to Nourish, Rejuvenate, and Transform Your Life / Sebastian Pole.
    pages cm
  Includes bibliographical references and index.
  ISBN 978-1-58394-671-8
  1. Medicine, Ayurvedic. 2. Traditional medicine—India. 3. Holistic medicine. I. Title.
  R606.P65 2013
  610—dc23
                        2013010028

1 2 3 4 5 6 7 8 9 C&C printing 18 17 16 15 14 13

CONTENTS

Introduction   6

❀ 1 Constitution   10
❀ 2 Nourishment   36
❀ 3 Cleansing   70
❀ 4 Rejuvenation   100
❀ 5 Strength and Stillness   134
❀ 6 Ecology   174
❀ 7 Relationship   204

The Pukka Pantry   230

Glossary   246
Selected Bibliography   248
Resources   249
Index   252
Acknowledgments   256

Welcome to *Discovering the True You with Ayurveda*. Writing this book has inspired me and I hope reading it will inspire you. *Discovering the True You* is for anyone interested in learning more about their health, their heart, their mind, the principles of Ayurveda, yoga, and herbal medicine.

I have tried to write an accessible book that you can use in your everyday life. To this end, I have kept images of my patients, my family, and anyone seeking vitality in my mind's eye while writing. My wish is that the book helps you comprehend your life on a deeper level and allows you to enjoy it more, because that is what Ayurveda is all about—finding a path to a state of authentic happiness.

I am no classical Ayurvedic doctor, or *vaidya*, as they are officially known. My training has been eclectic to say the least, but I have been fortunate enough to have had some inspiring teachers during my seven years' formal study of Ayurveda, Chinese medicine, the Western tradition of herbal medicine, and yoga. I have now seen so many incredible healings that I have an absolute belief that our wholeness can only flourish if we tend to all of our complex and multifaceted selves from many different angles. It's no good just taking chamomile for stress if you have some deep-set trauma in your life; you need massage, a support group, therapy, and meditation practice as well. You need a whole orchestra to really sing your life song.

Ayurveda is translated as "knowledge of life" and encompasses the idea of how to live wisely. In particular, it is the knowledge of how to live according to your unique and individual constitutional make up, placing the choices of how you exist firmly in your court. A description given in the *Charaka Samhita*, an early Ayurvedic text written in about 100bce, notes: "It is called Ayurveda because it tells us which substances, qualities and actions are life-enhancing, and which are not." From its ancient origins in India, Ayurveda has now spread all over the world. Its teaching uses a blend of herbal medicine, massage, nutrition, spiritual insight, practical experience, scientific analysis, and artistic creativity to guide us to a balanced and fulfilled lifestyle. At its root is its focus on the uniqueness of each individual. As such it is a universal system applicable to every individual living in any part of the world—personal medicine at its best.

Despite its apparent simplicity, Ayurveda is complete as a medical system because it deals not only with the treatment and management of specific diseases, but with health in all its aspects: physical health, mental balance, spiritual well-being, social welfare, relationships, environmental considerations, dietary habits, daily living trends, and seasonal variations in lifestyle. Ayurveda teaches respect for nature and appreciation of life by showing how we can empower ourselves as individuals. It understands that our own health cannot be considered as separate from that of our family, work, society, and planet. In other words, Ayurveda is a fully integrated health system.

Because Ayurveda is formed from interwoven ideas on nature and life, some of its teachings may appear prescriptive: how to live, when to get up, what to eat, and what not to eat. But actually Ayurveda has nothing to do with rules and restrictions; it is really about offering you insights into how you can fulfill your potential based on your own choice. And I have divided these insights into seven pathways, focusing on constitution, nourishment, cleansing, rejuvenation strength and stillness, ecology, and relationship. You can read them in any order you like, but approaching the chapters on constitution and nourishment first will equip you with some of the basic principles of Ayurveda.

Throughout, I have laid out a range of practices that are easy to use, effective, and fun. The benefits of many of these techniques are supported by a couple of thousand years of continuous use, scientific research, the realizations of many great healers, and my own clinical experience.

Think of discovering the true you not so much as a final destination to be reached, but as an ongoing journey. There will be twists and turns along the way, but as you learn to integrate Ayurveda in your daily existence you will be able to take more ownership over your life: your response to what crosses your path will begin to be your choice as opposed to what you feel you "should" do. Taking back responsibility for life is about laughing when there is joy, crying when there is sorrow, and being grateful for the wisdom-enhancing lessons—whether painful or pleasurable—that each day brings. This empowerment will allow you to embrace all of your life with integrity and love, expressing the real you in every thought, feeling, and action.

One way to have a fulfilling life is to be true to yourself and your values and this book is about that deep authenticity, which is why I've called it *Discovering the True You*. In India the word "pukka" sums up the attitude required for this journey. In Hindi, the word "pukka" means anything that is genuine, authentic, or real; in Britain, "pukka" is a colloquial word for being excellent, as in "It's totally pukka, mate." I just love the sound of the word: you pronounce it as though it has a long "h" on the end, as in "pukkah." Of course, the other reason that I love the word is that the company I set up in 2001, with my good friend and partner Tim Westwell, is called Pukka Herbs. As we would say in Britain, "We sell pukka herbs" and I have has the privilege of being involved in the sourcing of organically grown herbs and in making delicious herbal teas and remedies for over a decade now.

Ayurveda's time-honored system of health guides us along a path that leads us from the stresses and ills of life to a place of peace and health. It's not always easy, and it's certainly not an evolution that progresses in a single straight line, but the knowledge and understanding I have received in following its guidance have added immeasurably to the richness of my life.

This book is one that I will give to all of my patients as they forge their way to fulfillment. It's also one that I am going to read again and again, to remind myself of the things to which I aspire. But, ultimately, *Discovering the True You* is a book for you and I hope you find the guidance and inspiration to do just that.

With my blessings,

Sebastian Pole
Bath, UK
2013

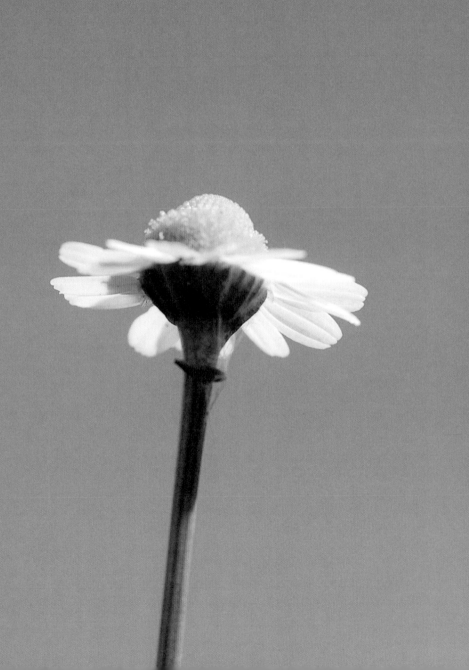

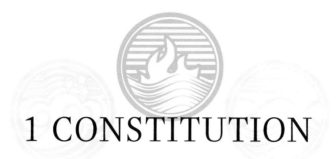

1 CONSTITUTION

"The three constitutions are wind (vata), fire (pitta), and water (kapha). They destroy or maintain the body, according to whether they are sick or healthy."
ASHTANGA HRIDAYA SAMHITA

We all want to be healthy so that we have the best chance to enjoy and fulfill our potential in life. But excellent health seems to be such a complicated subject that it is not always easy to know how to achieve this holy grail. Although at first it might appear to be an alien concept, understanding your constitution goes a long way in helping you to realize your perfect health. In Ayurveda your personal constitution is known as *prakriti*, which means "nature," as in your inherent genetic type. Ayurveda teaches us how to find out what our constitution is by observing who we are and how we feel. And this lesson is a very simple and enriching one. As you learn what your real nature is, you can live a truly authentic life—a life that suits you and allows your health to flourish.

WHAT IS HEALTH?

A healthy person is someone whose body, mind, and spirit are integrated as a unified whole. Although linguistically we commonly distinguish between our body and mind, in reality there is no difference: our body is filled with neurons that "think" and send messages, just as our mind works in a functional, "bodily" way, digesting, absorbing, and eliminating life's experiences. This idea of wholeness is represented by the term "body–mind" throughout the book.

For someone to be healthy, their hormonal, immune, and nervous systems should be integrated; these must work in a balanced synergy that is not overloaded or undernourished. A healthy person has constructive attitudes and positive approaches to opportunities and challenges, while still experiencing the mystery and wonder of life. A healthy person lives in a loving way within their environment and culture to optimize the vitality and potential of the whole. A healthy person feels joyful enough to dance to the radio at breakfast time.

The signs of optimum health include:

* a healthy appetite and a balanced desire for food without extreme cravings
* an appreciation of the flavor of food and feeling satisfied after eating
* good digestion without any signs of discomfort, belching, flatulence, or borborygmus (a wonderfully onomatopoeic word meaning "rumblings")
* a clear voice
* being free from any pain or discomfort
* proper functioning of the senses: effective and efficient hearing, feeling, seeing, tasting, and smelling
* a clear complexion
* regular elimination of feces, urine, and sweat
* the appropriate length and quality of sleep
* waking up and feeling positive
* constant energy with good stamina and ability to exercise
* enthusiasm for life
* youthfulness and slow aging
* balanced emotions: neither too happy with success nor too sad in times of difficulty
* being regularly compassionate, peaceful, loving, generous, and calm

DISCOVERING YOUR CONSTITUTION

Understanding your constitution is empowering. It gives you insight into who you are, how you should live, what you should eat, and how to get the most out of life. It brings you knowledge of yourself and what is best for you. It informs your choices and decisions.

Our constitution can be understood by viewing human beings as a microcosm of the macrocosm, much like in Gaia Theory, where our inner world mirrors the outer world (*see* Ecology, p.192). By noticing the different qualities of the natural world around you and within you, you can discover your own individual nature.

The language of nature

A good starting point is to define how we talk about our constitution. Having developed at a time when cultures were profoundly dependent on their environment, Ayurveda uses language derived from nature as a metaphor to describe and prescribe for our health. According to its teachings, the foundational elements of Ether (or Space), Air (or its more dynamic aspect, Wind), Fire, Water, and Earth are the building blocks that make up our physical world (*see* Ecology, p.178 for further discussion). We use adjectives to describe these elements as they appear in their different forms, which Ayurveda depicts as ten pairs of opposing qualities (known as *guna*s): hot, cold; heavy, light; dry, greasy; sharp, dull; rough, smooth; stable, mobile; soft, hard; liquid, solid; subtle, gross; slimy, non slimy. We routinely say, "It's a warm day," "The ground is wet," but this is also your language to describe yourself in sickness and in health: "My legs feel heavy," "My skin is dry and rough."

Whenever you are observing something, ask yourself about its particular qualities: is it hot or cold, wet or dry, light or heavy? Consider places and ecosystems: the Arizona desert, with its arid, sandy expanses, is "hot" and "dry," while the British countryside, with its lush green fields, is "cold" and "wet." Every disease has a typical blueprint, too: a fever is a "hot" and "dry" disease because you have a temperature and are thirsty, while a head cold is a "cold" and "damp" disease because you feel chilly and have a congested nose. Foods also have different qualities. Wheat products are heavy, wet, and cooling—think of a bread dough or cake batter: it is very sticky and moist. Spices are generally light, dry, and heating. Just chew on a chile and feel your mouth burn.

We will keep returning to these metaphorical adjectives throughout the book as we weave together the different parts of nature that make up our world and your constitutional balance.

THE THREE CONSTITUTIONAL TYPES (*DOSHAS*)

"Vata, pitta *and* kapha *move in the whole body producing good or ill effects upon the entire system, according to their normal or aggravated states. Their normal state is balance and their aggravated state is illness.*" *CHARAKA SAMHITA*

Although we are all beautifully unique, and there are as many constitutions as there are people, Ayurveda divides us into three main constitutional types, *vata, pitta,* and *kapha*, otherwise known as *dosha*s. The *dosha*s are qualities that influence all of the body's functions, from biological processes to thoughts and feelings. We all contain *vata, pitta,* and *kapha*, but it is their particular combination that makes us who we are. The division between the *dosha*s is the keystone to understanding Ayurveda, helping us determine and manage our genetic constitution, or *prakriti*. Understanding this very profound knowledge, passed down through at least 75 generations of Ayurvedic teachers, has the potential to change your life.

*Dosha*s, although present from birth, are not inert: they can change according to a variety of circumstances, such as what food we eat, whether the weather is hot or cold, how happy we are feeling, how late we go to bed. The literal meaning of the Sanskrit word *dosha* is "fault," because when circumstances cause a particular *dosha* to accumulate in excess, or to become aggravated, it can result in discomfort—the *dosha*s literally "overflow." We each have a threshold and when this is reached it causes a temporary imbalance in the *dosha*s known as *vikriti* (literally, "imbalanced"). If left unchecked, this imbalance becomes chronic and health problems start. Ayurveda spends a lot of its time teaching us how to remain within our threshold, and understanding the three *dosha*s will help you to do this.

It is common to be a combination of constitutional types: some people are pure *vata, pitta,* or *kapha*, but many are *vata-pitta, vata-kapha,* or *pitta-kapha* (the dominant quality is listed first), or—more rarely—an equal balance of all three, *vata-pitta-kapha. See* the *Pukka Practice* on p.32 to discover your genetic constitution (*prakriti*) and any current health imbalance (*vikriti*).

Like increases like (*samanya-vaisheshika*)

All of nature has qualities that impact on our own constitutional well-being. For example, if we are already a "hot" body type, and we live in the desert and eat lots of heating food, we will become too hot! This elucidates a fundamental Ayurvedic principle that like increases like, meaning that the qualities of our constitution can be added to by qualities that are similar to it. And, conversely, these qualities can be lessened by exposure to experiences, foods, and environments that are opposite to it. This principle of "like increasing like" and "opposites balancing opposites" is central to understanding how Ayurvedic treatments work, and you will be finding out a lot more about it as you read on. Deep down, we know it already—it is part of our human intuition. We just need to tune into it and translate this knowledge into a language that we can understand and utilize.

VATA
—dry, cold, light, mobile, subtle, rough, irregular

Vata is the principle of communication and movement. It is the messenger, regulating the nervous and immune systems and overseeing the input-output functions in our body. As such, it is responsible for all movement in the body: the flow of breath, the expression of speech, circulation of blood, elimination of wastes, menstruation, giving birth. It moves the diaphragm, muscles, and limbs and also stimulates the intellect.

All of these functions illustrate how the *vata* constitution or *dosha* is comprised mainly of the qualities of Space and Wind. Wind moves through space; you can't see space or the wind but you can feel a cool breeze on your skin. *Vata* is the Wind element that is held within the vast expanse of Space, such as our atmosphere, a hollow cave, or our intestines. *Vata* is an expression of the inherent nature of these foundational elements; like a chill wind, *vata* is cold, light, rough, mobile, irregular, subtle, clear, dry, and astringent. When *vata* manifests, we experience these qualities in how we feel physically and emotionally, perhaps with dry skin, poor circulation, or low body weight.

Like a current of electricity, *vata* is busy: it is responsible for regulating all electrical impulses in the body–mind, carrying information in and out. In fact, without *vata* the other *dosha*s are inert. As it says in the Ayurvedic literature, "*Pitta* is lame, *kapha* is lame. They go wherever the wind (*vata*) takes them, just like the clouds." When in balance, *vata* brings comfortable movement, regular breathing, a consistent appetite, normal excretion of wastes, positive enthusiasm, healthy desire, good energy, a calm mind, and inspirational creativity.

However, because of its dynamic nature, aggravated *vata* is often involved in the movement of disease around the body. It carries arthritis to the joints, acne to the skin, and fatty deposits to the arteries. In the body, *vata*'s "home" is below the belly button, especially in the colon. It can also occupy the bladder, thighs, ears, bones, and the sense of touch. Problems in these parts of the body are often (but not always) to do with *vata* being out of balance.

Vata is also creative. *Vata* types are inspirational, always full of ideas. They are often geniuses, artists, or inventors. But with this creative flare and "airy" nature come some irregularities. They have long and irregularly shaped limbs, curly hair, and angular features. They move like the wind, are impulsive, and love change. For more details on the wonderful manifestations of *vata*, *see* chart on the next page.

FEATURE	*VATA* CHARACTERISTICS
SOUNDS	
Voice	Dry, hoarse, high-pitched, or quiet
	Fast talker, jumps from subject to subject
Other noises	Cracking joints, burping, a bit windy
WHAT IT FEELS LIKE	
Pulse	Cold, hard, thin, fast, irregular
Skin	Cold and dry, especially hands, knees, nose, feet, abdomen
APPEARANCE	
Physical frame	Very tall or short, thin, delicately slender
	Knobbly knees and elbows
Weight	Low weight
	Finds it difficult to put on weight
Skin	Dry, rough, chapped, cracks on hands and feet
	Veins visible through skin
	Pale lips, nail beds and skin; blue when very cold
	Tans easily
Hair	Dry, thin, curly, wiry, dark, frizzy
	Scant hair over body
Nails	Dry, rough, irregular length and shape
	May have white spots and ridges; may be brittle
Eyes	Gray, dark blue, or dark brown
	Small in relation to head and can feel dry
	Eyebrows thin, regular in shape
Tongue	Thin, small, dry, cracked, and thin
	Pale in color with a white or black coating
Smell	Hardly any body odor
	Rarely sweats
HABITS	
Digestion	Variable, irregular, and "nervous" appetite
	Can suffer from bloating and flatulence
	Constipation, dry stools, irregular bowel movements
Sleep	Irregular pattern, light to very deep, averaging 4–7 hours; can suffer from insomnia
	Prone to sleepwalking and -talking; teeth-grinding common
	Wakes early, feels a bit "burned-out"
	Rarely remembers dreams, usually about motion
	Prefers a soft bed with heavy cover

Energy levels	Erratic, comes in waves
	Bad managers of vitality, often try to sustain energy with stimulants
Sex drive	Varies. Avid fantasizers
	Intensely passionate, then needs rest
	Can have weaker fertility
Temperature needs	Easily feels cold, wears lots of warm clothes
	Likes hot drinks and food
	Likes a warm and humid climate
	Dislikes cold, dry, and windy weather
Mood	When balanced, is creative and inspirational
	If imbalanced, can be a bit anxious and fearful
TIMES	
Day	Prevalent very early morning and early afternoon (often the windiest time of day); predominantly 3–7am and 3–7pm
Season	The change of the seasons, especially spring and fall
Age	Later life, above the age of 50 (older people are full of wisdom and, like *vata*, are thinner, drier, lighter)
FAMOUS PEOPLE	Mahatma Gandhi, Bob Dylan, Victoria Beckham, Kylie Minogue

When *vata* is out of balance

If *vata* is imbalanced there may be a variety of symptoms, depending on whether there is too much or too little *vata*. With an excess of *vata* you may lose weight, experience piercing pains or spasms, rigidity, numbness, cracking joints, dry skin, dehydration, an astringent taste in the mouth, dark discolorations of the skin and bodily excretions, dizziness, painful or scanty periods, and insomnia. Too little *vata* and you may feel sluggish and lazy, and, more extremely, suffer from confusion, deliriousness, and loss of consciousness. *Vata* diseases, such as osteoporosis, arthritis, or Alzheimer's, tend to increase later in life.

While *vata* types can have natural creative flare, an excess of *vata* can make you increasingly fearful, anxious, nervous, lonely, and depressed. How many great artists have been almost too sensitive for our world? Not enough *vata* can create a lack of enthusiasm or the desire to speak. The *dosha*'s light, scattered, and erratic nature means that *vata* types need to be wary of circumstances, places, and people that make them feel insecure and frightened.

You can balance *vata*'s cold, airy tendencies by increasing its opposing qualities: more warmth, moisture, and earthiness, and reducing those experiences that are light, cold, or dry. For more details on how to balance *vata*, *see* Cleansing, p.90.

PITTA
—hot, sharp, penetrating, slightly oily, greasy, fast, irritable

Pitta is the principle of passion and metabolism. It is the manager, regulating the information that *vata* has brought into the body through efficient handling of potential energy. It therefore controls digestion and metabolism, as well as overseeing the cellular generation of energy.

Pitta's functions show that this *dosha* is made up of the qualities of Fire and Water, the regulatory elements in nature. This seemingly contradictory combination actually works in complementary fashion: *pitta* exists as water or oil in the body, preserving the tissues from the destructive aspect of fire. Just think of the moist lining in the stomach protecting it from fiery and potentially corrosive digestive juices. Like a raging volcano, *pitta* is pungent, hot, penetrating, oily, sharp, liquid, spreading, and sour. If *pitta* is high you can feel these qualities in the body when you are hot, have oily skin, or are burning with hunger.

Because of its hot nature, *pitta*'s primary function is transformation. It is the force of metabolic activity in the body, controlling the heartbeat, hormone levels, body temperature, visual perception, hunger, thirst, and skin quality. *Pitta* is also specifically responsible for the function of the liver, the secretion of bile, and digestion in the stomach and small intestine. On the mental level it plays a role in understanding and in digesting sensory impressions. *Pitta*'s main "home" in the body is in the small intestine, but it also resides in the eyes, blood, sweat glands, stomach, lymph, and in the emotional aspect of the heart (*see* Rejuvenation, p.112). When in balance, you experience a healthy appetite and thirst, balanced production of hormones and enzymes, intelligence, courage, flexibility, a healthy complexion, and strong eyesight.

Pitta is full of vitality. *Pitta* people are charming and charismatic leaders who love to be the center of attention. In fact, they are great fun to be around as they are so dynamic and colorful. They are good planners and get things done. For more details on the wonderful manifestations of *pitta see* the chart opposite.

FEATURE	*PITTA* CHARACTERISTICS
SOUNDS	
Voice	Loud, sharp, precise
	Focused, persuasive, dominating
Other noises	Sighing
WHAT IT FEELS LIKE	
Pulse	Warm, soft, regular, wiry, strong
Skin	Hot flushes, warm hands, moist skin
APPEARANCE	
Physical frame	Medium, balanced build with defined muscles
	Athletic body
Weight	Average weight for build
	Maintains a balanced weight
Skin	Delicate but easily irritated and often red; flushes easily
	Intolerant to sun
	Tendency for freckles, moles, rashes, and acne
Hair	Straight, blond, brown, or red
	Often early graying with early balding
Nails	Soft, strong, pliable
	Deep red nail beds
Eyes	Light color
	Sharp, piercing, and sensitive to light
	Balanced eyebrows and lashes
Tongue	Medium-sized tongue, often with a pointed red tip
	Bright red or purple in color with a yellowish coating
Smell	Strong and pungent smell
	Sweats profusely in hot weather
HABITS	
Digestion	Fierce appetite, easily irritable if hungry
	Can suffer from heartburn and acidity
	Rarely constipated but can have loose stools
Sleep	Sleeps well, averaging 4–7 hours
	Often night owls
	May have intense, colorful dreams involving action
	Prefers a firm bed with few covers
Energy levels	Good energy levels that are regular and consistent
	Can become addicted to the "buzz" of working
Sex drive	Strong sexual appetite
	Good fertility

Temperature needs	Feels warm and wears thin, light clothes
	Prefers cool drinks and some raw food
	Likes cool and mild weather
	Dislikes a hot and humid climate
Mood	When balanced, positive and playful
	When imbalanced, aggressive and overly competitive
	Goes for what they want and are irritable if they don't get it
TIMES	
Day	Midday (the warmest part of the day); predominantly 11am–3pm and 11pm–3am, and especially at midnight
Season	Late spring and summer
Age	Midlife, between 16–50 years of age: the time to organize, manage, work hard, build a career, have a family
FAMOUS PEOPLE	Marilyn Monroe, Tony Blair, Madonna, David Beckham

When *pitta* is out of balance

Signs of an increase in *pitta* include an aversion to heat, a sour or bitter taste in the mouth, loose stools, and yellow, green, and red discolorations in the eyes, skin, and bodily excretions. You may have heartburn, high blood pressure, a fever, skin rashes, hot flushes, and suffer from fainting. Too little *pitta* results in increased signs of *vata* (*see* p.15) and *kapha* (*see* opposite), poor digestion, pallor, and coldness. *Pitta* imbalances tend to increase with the onset of puberty and carry on through midlife, resulting in acne, menstrual or hormonal irregularities, hyperacidity, heart problems, or inflammations.

Emotionally, an imbalanced *pitta* manifests as anger, frustration, and irritation, often as a result of repressed emotions. *Pitta* people are archetypal critics, quick to judge others but quietly harshest on themselves. Being extremely competitive, they are often plagued by jealousy. To balance the "intense" nature of *pitta*, try to find opposing qualities of calm, coolness, compassion, and moderation. For more details, *see* Cleansing, p.90.

KAPHA
—cold, wet, heavy, stable, solid, unctuous, slow

Kapha is the principle of love and structure, and is responsible for stability and moisture in the body (*kapha* literally means "that which flourishes in water"). *Kapha* takes charge of the storage of the energy that *vata* has brought in and that *pitta* has managed, in the form of fats in the cell membrane and carbohydrates in the cell wall. This helps to give lubrication, structure, and form to the whole body.

The *kapha dosha* is a combination of the Earth and Water elements. Just as earth is moistened by reviving water, its dry dust forming binding mud, *kapha* literally holds the body together by moistening the "earthen" structures of the tissues and skin. Like a meandering river, *kapha* is slow, heavy, cool, dense, soft, oily, sticky, cloudy, liquid, and sweet. It is cohesive, gives shape and form, and aids growth and development. Its fluid qualities regulate the experience of taste and smell, the cerebrospinal fluid and white matter in the brain, the synovial fluid that nourishes the joints, the lubrication of the lungs and heart, and the protective lining of the stomach. It relates to phlegm in the body, and *kapha* types often suffer from mucus congestion. Its primary "home" is the stomach and it also resides in the chest, heart, throat, head, pancreas, stomach, lymph, fat, nose, and tongue. When in balance it gives strength, solidity, protection, and endurance.

Kapha people are full of love and compassion. You can always rely on a *kapha* person in a time of need—they are very loyal and devout. They are your best friend, are very solid, and give great hugs. For more details on the wonderful manifestations of *kapha, see* chart on the next page.

FEATURE	*KAPHA* CHARACTERISTICS
SOUNDS	
Voice	Moist, soft, deep, calm
	Speaks slowly
Other noises	Heavy footfall, tendency to snore
WHAT IT FEELS LIKE	
Pulse	Cool, strong, slow, regular
Skin	Regular circulation, cool skin that feels damp
APPEARANCE	
Physical frame	Big bones, a stocky, solid body
	Wide hips, shoulders, short, stubby fingers
Weight	Tends to excess body weight
	Difficulty in losing weight
Skin	Healthy, thick, oily, smooth
	Burns in the sun but soon tans
Hair	Often brown, abundant, thick, wavy, can be oily
	Can have a very hairy body
Nails	Large, thick, strong, symmetrical
	White, soft
Eyes	Brown
	Large and oval with white sclera
	Bushy eyebrows, thick lashes
Tongue	Thick, swollen, flabby, often with teeth marks
	Pale with a thick white coating
Smell	Moderate, sweet aroma
	Sweats easily with exercise
HABITS	
Digestion	Stable appetite, slow digestion
	Loves food, may comfort eat
	Regular but sluggish bowel movements
Sleep	Heavy sleep of 8 or more hours
	Difficulty in waking; calm, smooth, and emotional dreams
	Prefers a soft bed and medium amount of covers
Energy levels	Solid, consistent levels
	Reluctant to expend energy
	Would rather drive than walk
Sex drive	Steady sexual appetite
	Very loving and compassionate
	Excellent fertility

Temperature needs	Feels cool and wears soft, comfy clothes
	Likes warm food and warm drinks
	Likes warm but dry climate
Mood	Dislikes the climate when it is too cold or too hot
	When balanced, supportive and strong
	When imbalanced, greedy and lazy
TIMES	
Day	Morning (a damp and dewy time); predominantly 7–11am and 7–11pm
Season	Winter and early spring
Age	Childhood (children are soft, loving, and cuddly)
FAMOUS PEOPLE	Winston Churchill, Muhammad Ali, Oprah Winfrey, Catherine Zeta-Jones

When *kapha* is out of balance

Signs of too much *kapha* include excess mucus and salivation, sticky phlegm, a wet cough, itching, coldness, heaviness, stagnation, congestion, growths, cysts, tumors, dull pain, edema, sluggish digestion, excessive desire to sleep, sweet and salty tastes in the mouth, and thick and white discharges. If *kapha* is out of balance then this may manifest in heart problems, diabetes, high cholesterol or in being overweight. Too little *kapha* and there will be signs of *vata* increase, for example, cracking joints, dryness, dizziness, and weight loss. *Kapha* problems, such as coughs and glue ear, often develop in childhood, a time of growth. *Kapha*'s inherent role in the storing of energy can mean that, on an emotional level, *kapha* people have a tendency to hold on to and accumulate both people and things— they can be a bit greedy and possessive.

To balance some of this *dosha*'s tendency to "hold on," *kapha* types can try to let go of more in life, increase the amount of movement they do, undertake more stimulating activities, share more, and clear out their cupboards more regularly. For more details on how to balance *kapha*, *see* Cleansing, p.91.

PUKKA PERSPECTIVES

THE GENETIC HERETIC

The paradigm of modern medicine is to dissect the whole and try to determine our entirety by studying its parts. Recent scientific discoveries have seemingly reduced us to the symmetrical, swirling double-helix bond of DNA. But in reducing nature to its smallest components, what we are left with is incredible detail but a partial truth. A well-known Indian story says that it is a bit like a blind person trying to describe an elephant by touching only its trunk, tail, or legs. While the existence of DNA may be scientifically true, therapeutically valuable, and even aesthetically beautiful, it is not indicative of the whole picture.

In addition, this current approach to medicine is disempowering: it tends to take the responsibility for health away from the individual and put it in someone else's hands, such as a "doctor's" or a "national health system." Which is not to say that doctors are not responsible individuals, but rather that the science is so complex, the definition of disease so reductionist, and the drugs so alien, that individuals cannot take charge of their own health. Moreover, our current "one pill for one disease" system does not empower the person to understand the interconnectivity of their whole being.

The holistic approach

What distinguishes Ayurvedic practice from modern medical practice is that it is concerned with the connection between things, such as between us and our environment, our digestion and the food we eat, our emotions and our relationships, and how they all contribute to our health. To put this notion into a more fitting genetic language, Ayurveda is interested in our constitutional phenotypes (the results we can observe when an individual interacts with their environment) rather than our human genotypes (the genetic constitution of an individual).

Ayurveda teaches that disease is primarily due to an imbalance in the inner processes of the body–mind, resulting in an imbalance in your constitutional tendency: too much heat, cold, wetness, or dryness. This is different from the functional view of illness that regards organs in isolation from each other and germs as sole causes of disease. This tension between different schools of medicine was made famous by the nineteenth-century debates between the French scientists Claude Bernard and Louis Pasteur, concerning their respective "inner terrain" versus the "external germ" theories. Which is more relevant to vitality, they argued: the health of the body and its internal resistance (the *milieu intérieur*, or homeostasis, as it is now known), or the strength of the invading microbe? On his deathbed Pasteur supposedly relented: "The terrain is everything, the germ is nothing." However, the "germ theory" of medicine persisted and the rest is pharmaceutical history, as it developed into a cornerstone of modern medicine and the wellspring of the drug industry. Whatever Pasteur actually said, germs do play an important role in numerous diseases, of course, but so does the inner resistance of the person they flourish in. And it is this essential part of health that has largely been forgotten by modern medical interventions.

By contrast, Ayurveda understands both the potential risks of invading organisms and the value of eradicating a harmful assault as well as perceiving that disease is caused by the whole system being out of balance, not simply by an isolated bacteria or hormone. Its approach seeks to address this imbalance by initially educating people in how to prevent disease from happening in the first place, and then by addressing the *whole person* so that effective and complete healing on a physical, mental, emotional, and spiritual level can take place—a healing so deep that even our genetic potential can be transformed. And it is this perspective of the whole that we need to include in order to fulfill our health potential.

THE ROOTS OF GOOD HEALTH

Ayurveda recommends integrating your "being" into your "doing," so that your life is your "practice." Whether your focus is on health, wealth, joy, or spiritual growth, how you lead your life becomes an expression of who you really are. It is easy to be "good" in the gym or when sitting in meditation, but being able to bring your intention for how you want to live into your daily life is a special skill. It needs practice to be successful. In my experience, it is an ongoing process which is made easier by having simple daily routines that keep your unique constitutional blend of *vata*, *pitta,* and *kapha* refreshed and rejuvenated and your intention focused. Unless you are a saint or have an entourage of assistants, there is no way that you can follow them all every day. I certainly don't—life is just too busy. However, even just doing what you can will have a huge impact on your life. Introduce the routines slowly and, before you know it, your days will be filled with healing habits.

 Getting up

When you can, follow the seasons, rising later in the darker mornings of winter and earlier in the lighter mornings of summer. Try to make the time for a peaceful moment of reflection before you launch into your day. Because of the principle of "like increasing like" (*see* box p.14), sleeping into *kapha* time (7–11am) causes problems such as tiredness, sluggish liver, poor appetite, slow bowels, and muzzy-headedness (although you can overcome this by being active thereafter). However, people who are exhausted, ill, young children, the elderly, and pregnant or breast-feeding women do not need to get up so early—they require more rest.

 Elimination

It is best to move your bowels first thing in the morning, so drink some hot water with fresh lemon juice on rising to awaken the digestive system, flush out accumulated toxins, and get your bowels going. Hot water or herbal tea are better than black tea or coffee, as they are gentle to digest, stimulate your digestive energy, and relax your bowels. If your system needs more encouragement or if you are constipated, take a mild digestive tonic such as triphala (*see* The Pukka Pantry), a mixture of three antioxidant-packed, bowel-nourishing fruits, in the morning and evening.

 Oral hygiene

Ayurveda considers that astringent, bitter, and pungent flavors (*see* Nourishment, pp.51–3) are the best for helping to clear bacteria from the mouth and reducing inflammation in the gums. A toothpaste containing myrrh, peppermint, propolis, and/or neem meets these requirements and has additional circulation-enhancing properties. Flossing your teeth dislodges bacteria from the gums. You can also clean your tongue with a tongue scraper, which helps to dispel bad breath and stimulates your digestive system via the gastric reflex. Finally, gargle with warm water to clear your throat.

 ## Cleaning your body

I can't even consider starting my day without a wash. It makes me feel fresh and awake. Use warm water for *vata* and *kapha*, cool or cold water if you are a hot *pitta* type. You can then follow this with three simple practices known as the three "N"s; *neti, nasya,* and *netra shodhana*, or nasal wash, nasal oiling, and eye cleansing. These remarkable yogic cleansing practices sound slightly bizarre but are exceptional for maintaining the immunity of the entire nasal and eye region.

For a nasal wash, fill a *neti* pot (a bit like a small teapot, and found in most yoga centers) with a salt water solution (1 teaspoon salt added to some warm water). Tilt your head to one side, place the spout in the upper nostril, and gently pour the water up your nose so that it comes out of the other open nostril. This saline solution draws mucus out of the sinuses by osmosis as it washes over the mucous membrane lining of the nostrils. Follow with some rapid breathing in and out of the nose, forcefully expelling the air, to dry the nostrils.

For the ultimate Ayurvedic start to your day, next put a couple of drops of medicated nasal oil into your nose to keep the sinuses clear and to awaken your mind. Often called "*nasya* oil," it is made from sesame oil blended with decongesting and mind-awakening herbs like vacha, brahmi, and turmeric (*see* The Pukka Pantry), and is ideal for protecting the nasal membranes against the dryness of the colder seasons.

If you are having a super-cleansing day, wash your eyes using eyedrops (*netra shodhana*). I like to use a couple of drops of organic rosewater, either straight into the eye or on a cotton wool pad as a wipe.

 ## Oil massage

One of the guiding principles behind Ayurvedic medicine, massage can be a wonderful part of your daily regime, as it is cleansing, nourishing, relaxing, and balancing: it cleans the body, emolliates and nourishes the skin, regulates the constitution, and moves displaced *dosha*s back to the digestive tract. Specifically, it helps protect you from the degenerative diseases of old age, such as arthritis, while also promoting sound sleep and—so the sages tell us—good vision and a long life. You don't need a professional to do this—it's easy enough to give yourself a massage. I do a brief one most days using sesame oil and try to do a more thorough, full-body oil massage every week. For more on massage *see* Strength and Stillness, p.170.

 ## Exercise

Ayurveda has a view that people should practice stimulating exercise up to the point of producing a mild sweat and not beyond. It also recommends that we should exercise only for as long as we can comfortably breathe through our nostrils. This "nostril only" breathing is as relevant to your yoga postures as to any metabolic exercise: as you learn to control your breath, your fitness and energy will really increase.

When exercising, choose an activity that is appropriate for you. Pay attention to your body and your breath. Do not overdo any repetitive exercise that stresses one specific part of the body excessively (for example, jogging, skipping, weightlifting), especially if you are a thin *vata* type—for you, a yoga class or a brisk walk in the park would be more beneficial. *Pitta* people can do more metabolic exercise as they are natural athletes. It doesn't have to be a standard workout at your local gym— something that is fun and creative will do just as well. *Kapha* types can do even more metabolic exercise and, in fact, more sweating is good for them. Try trampolining, skipping, or hula-hooping.

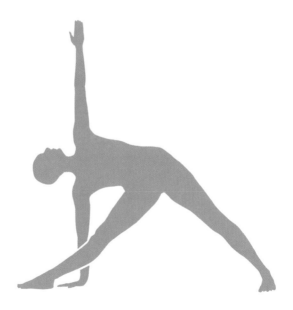

A simple exercise It is not always easy to exercise every day but try to take some time to stretch your limbs to invigorate circulation, feed your cells, and remove tension. Do this practice at any time of day.

Stand firmly with your legs hip-width apart. Feel your weight sink into the ground. Ground your heels to the floor, relax your shoulders, soften your belly. Take a deep breath in and let a long breath out. Now start to bounce on your heels. As the weight of your body taps the ground, shake all the tension and stress from yourself. Breathe it out. Bounce, bounce, bend your knees, shake your arms, wiggle your hands and fingers, roll your head, loosen your hair. Bend forward at the hips slightly. Breathe out. Keep shaking. Then lean back and arch your back a little. Keep bouncing gently. Carry on for a few minutes and then stop. Feel your feet sinking into the ground, bend your knees, relax your pelvis, drop your shoulders, and close your eyes. And breathe. You should be firmly back in your body now.

Some dietary advice
- ❀ Have a light breakfast of nourishing grains: porridge or rice pudding
- ❀ Chew cardamom, fennel or anise throughout the day to keep your digestion stimulated (*see* next page)
- ❀ If you can, have your main meal in middle of the day, when the solar energy and inner fire are strongest
- ❀ Eat warm food as it is easier to digest; avoid cold and refrigerated food
- ❀ Avoid stale or processed food – it has little nutritional value and tastes rubbish
- ❀ Don't eat too much or too little – your digestion doesn't like extremes
- ❀ If you are not truly hungry, don't eat, or just have a light soup
- ❀ Take time to enjoy your food – it will taste better and be easier to digest
- ❀ Drink warm herbal teas throughout the day because they encourage your digestive fire, taste good and have many health benefits

 ## Meditation
Despite the popular view of it as serious and a tiny bit scary, meditation can be simple, relaxing, and deeply rewarding. And it can be practiced by anybody, anywhere, at any time. Nevertheless there are some basic skills to be learned which, once mastered, can help to raise awareness, give clarity of mind, and create inner peace. For more on the important technique of meditation, *see* Strength and Stillness, p.164.

 ## Eating
Eating should make you happy, and leave you nourished and satisfied. Ayurveda says that we should eat until the stomach is half-full of food and one-quarter full of water, with the remainder left for digestive energy to circulate. This is not always easy, as you can't actually see what is going on, so just be aware of how you feel as you are eating. Tuning into this inner intelligence can help guide you about

appropriate quantities of food, as well as what you can digest well. Without doubt my greatest lesson in health has been to follow and learn from my digestion. While my habits are far from perfect, this awareness helps me stay in touch with what and how I am eating in relation to what I need. This is delicious education. For specific details on the appropriate foods for your constitution, *see* Nourishment, p.64.

✳ Digestive stimulation

In order to act efficiently your digestive system often needs some stimulation before a meal. As your digestion can be metaphorically understood as a fire (*see* Nourishment, p.44), you can "stoke" it with stimulating, fiery spices, which accords with the Ayurvedic principle of "like increases like." So before each meal nibble on some fresh ginger or other warming spice (*see* box above), or take an Ayurvedic herbal digestive such as trikatu (*see* The Pukka Pantry).

✳ Lifestyle

Work is a large part of our lives. We have to be practical, pay the bills, and live in society—but there is always a choice. Try to organize your life so that you can follow a wholesome occupation that has some positive impact. This doesn't necessarily mean retiring to the monastery or only doing charitable work (although that might be right for you). It means doing something that promotes the welfare of your family, your community, society, and the environment, while including you and your hopes and dreams as much as you can. By doing a job that serves the whole, you are creating a positive circle of benevolence. And if life turns out to be not quite so ideal, then "it's not what you do but the way that you do it" that counts.

Know your local environment and climate intimately and adapt your daily lifestyle accordingly. If it's cold and wet make sure that your diet and clothes are warm and do not exacerbate the inherent dampness; it's a good idea to hold back on heavy, mucus-forming foods and don't go running in a skimpy top that exposes your belly and lower back—this is a one-way ticket to getting a cold. On the other hand, if it's hot and dry, eat moistening and cooling foods and don't go running at all; keep cool and relax. The important thing is to make sure that you regulate your lifestyle in accordance with your own personal daily needs.

THINKING AND FEELING YOUR WAY

"While resting in the spirit, the mind, pure and stable, shines as a lamp shines: with a bright flame from within the lantern."
CHARAKA SAMHITA

What we think is who we become. Consider the first verse of the Dhammapada, a text expressing the words of the Buddha: "We are what we think. All that we are arises with our thoughts. Mental phenomena are preceded by the mind, ruled by thought, made of mind. If you speak or act with a corrupted heart, then suffering follows you—just like the wheel of the cart follows the ox that pulls it ... If you speak or act with a calm, bright heart, then happiness follows you, like a shadow that never leaves." The truth of this verse is clear: as we think, so we become. Ayurvedic wisdom says that our waking consciousness rests in the heart. Experiencing how your mind lives in your heart is central to understanding how your feelings and emotions affect your experience of wholeness. For more on this important concept *see* Rejuvenation, p.114.

Ayurveda is a holistic system of medicine that sees the different dimensions of spirit-consciousness-mind-body as one continuum—that is one of the reasons why it is so powerful. It believes that consciousness condenses into mind before solidifying into the physical body. Hence our mind is the pivot between our conscious spiritual life and our physical one. Here, "mind" is a general term used to describe the part of us containing our thoughts, feelings, memory, intellect, perception, and will. Like a mirror, it reflects the brilliance of pure consciousness, which emanates from our spirit onto our intellect. It literally lights up our life. You need a clean mirror if you are going to get a clear view of consciousness.

Have you ever noticed how your mind can feel light and clear or foggy and muzzy, depending on what you've been going through? Our mind is the melting pot of our experiences, and the quality of the mental "broth" is a reflection of what goes in and what we do with it. And here lies your choice. What goes into your mind and how you choose to respond to it is the decisive factor in determining your health and happiness. This means that our state and quality of mind are integrally connected with disease and how we can deal with it. One of the main causes of disease is "mental seeds"—habits that no longer serve you—that are allowed to germinate and fester into a web of unhealthy patterns. The reverse is also true: healing thoughts can often initiate the cure of disease, engendering healthy habits and holistic living. While the cause of these unhealthy habits is not always easily identifiable, being aware of our constitutional tendencies will help point us in the right direction, and bring us closer to having an illuminated heart and mind. For a detailed discussion on the nature of the mind, *see* Strength and Stillness, p137.

PUKKA PRACTICE

DETERMINING YOUR CONSTITUTIONAL HEALTH

The following questionnaire will help you identify your genetically inherited constitutional type, or *prakriti*, and your current state of health. Firstly, answer the questions according to how you have been most consistently throughout your life. When you know which combination of *dosha*s you are, you can answer the questions again, focusing on the state of your health as it is today, your *vikriti*. After you have determined both your genetic constitution and which imbalances you are currently suffering from, you can start to follow a diet and lifestyle that suits you and will help you achieve optimum health. While this checklist will give you a good idea, to determine your constitution fully or for help with treating any chronic or serious health issues it is best to see a qualified Ayurvedic practitioner or herbalist (*see* Resources, p.250).

Tick the characteristics that *most* describe you.
(As many of us are a combination of *dosha*s, often more than one answer will apply. Choose any that are appropriate for you.)

Physical characteristics

1 How would you describe your body frame and weight?
a) Thin, irregular, prominent bones; low weight or underweight.
b) Medium, balanced bones; balanced, evenly maintained weight.
c) Large, solid bones; heavy or overweight.

2 What is your skin like?
a) Dry, cold, rough, thin, and dark, with cold hands and feet.
b) Moist, warm, smooth, oily, and rosy, fair with freckles and easily irritated.
c) Soft, cool, damp, thick, and pale.

3 How much do you sweat?
a) Hardly at all.
b) Profusely.
c) Moderately and consistently.

4 What is your hair like?
a) Dry, thin, dark, curly, knotted, and brittle, with split ends.
b) Oily, straight, blond/red/gray, or bald.
c) Oily, lustrous, thick, wavy, and brown.

5 What best describes your facial features?
a) Pointed, irregular nose and long nostrils, with thin, dry, and cracked lips.
b) Straight, roman nose, with deep red, moist, and soft lips.
c) Large, round nose and wide nostrils, with large, thick lips.

6 How would you describe your bodily features?
a) Small, slim hips; flat and deficient abdomen; thin legs with knobbly knees.
b) Medium hips; firm and moderate abdomen; medium-sized legs.
c) Large hips; soft, full, and large abdomen; strong, large legs.

7 What is your menstrual cycle like (women only)?
a) Irregular, mild, scanty flow, with clots, intense cramps, and dark color, and a tendency toward PMS and tearfulness.
b) Regular, heavy, long bleed, bright red color, medium cramps, and bad PMS and irritability.
c) Regular and easy, with dull cramps, water retention, and mild PMS.

Mind and emotions

1 How would you describe your sleep?
a) Disturbed. You're a light sleeper and often suffer from insomnia.
b) Good. Restful and you don't need much sleep.
c) Deep. You're a heavy sleeper and you sleep for long periods of time.

2 You've been set a team project. Which best describes your character in the group?
a) You're the creative one, full of wonderful and sometimes radical ideas, but when it comes to meetings you find yourself daydreaming and thinking about what you're doing at the weekend rather than taking notes.
b) You've written the project plan, organized the meetings, prepared immaculate handouts but if your ideas are criticized, you feel infuriated.
c) You're reliable, you do all the work you need to do, but it takes a lot of time and effort to complete the tasks.

3 You have an exam coming up. Which of these best describes how you prepare?
a) You cram in the study at the last minute. You just about remember what you need to for the next day but you'll forget it all by next week.
b) You have a meticulous study schedule, you've given yourself plenty of time to revise and you remember every detail.
c) It takes you ages to remember anything, but once you do, you never forget.

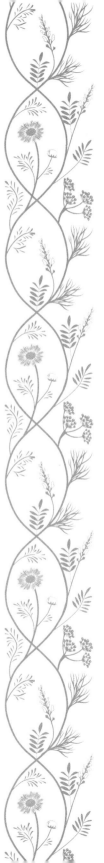

4 **You're at a party and someone is flirting outrageously with your partner. How do you react?**

- a) You feel insecure and anxious but you probably won't confront your partner.
- b) You turn into the green-eyed monster, the vol-au-vents are flying and you end up having a huge argument.
- c) You know you have nothing to worry about and you carry on having a great night with your friends.

Digestion

1 **Is your appetite:**

- a) Variable. You like to graze all day and pick at bits as and when you fancy.
- b) Regular. You like to eat at particular times but when you're hungry it's intense and you can't focus until you've had some food.
- c) Steady. You enjoy relaxed meals and take your time over your food.

2 **Is your thirst:**

- a) Variable. You generally prefer hot drinks.
- b) Regular. You're often thirsty and generally prefer cool drinks.
- c) Low. You rarely get thirsty.

3 **Would you consider your digestion and bowel movements to be:**

- a) Irregular. You're often bloated, gassy, or constipated. You always get constipated when you stay away from home.
- b) Regular as clockwork. You have a fast metabolism, evacuate your bowels everyday but can suffer from acidity or heartburn.
- c) Sluggish. You have a slow metabolism and sluggish bowels.

General health and energy

1 **What do you often suffer from?**

- a) Anxiety, insomnia, and nervous problems.
- b) Inflammation, bleeding problems, and skin problems.
- c) Mucus, congestion, and chest or heart problems.

2 **If you get ill, do you:**

- a) Get acute symptoms that start all of a sudden and then make a quick recovery.
- b) Suffer from fevers and sweating.
- c) Take a while to get an illness that then lingers for some time.

3 **What is your energy like? Do you:**

- a) Have extremes of energy that can be used up very quickly, leaving you exhausted.
- b) Have consistent energy and know how to pace yourself.
- c) Take a while to get going but then have excellent stamina.

4 How do you manage your weight?
a) You find it difficult to gain weight.
b) You have been able to maintain a regular weight throughout your life.
c) You find it very easy to put on weight.

5 What is your sex life like?
a) You have an erratic sexual appetite but are quickly aroused and have low fertility.
b) You have a passionate sexual appetite and good fertility.
c) You have a regular appetite, good stamina, and excellent fertility.

6 You're on vacation, it's 86 degrees in the shade. Which of the following best describes you?
a) You love the heat and are a sun worshipper. You go brown really easily.
b) You find the heat unbearable, you feel agitated, and all you want to do is stay in the pool. You can burn easily or get prickly heat rashes.
c) You don't mind the heat but prefer to take it easy and relax all day in the shade.

Your results

Now count up the number of "a"s, "b"s, and "c"s.

If your answers are mostly "a"s, you are predominantly *vata*; "b" corresponds to *pitta*; "c" indicates *kapha*. You will probably find that you are a combination of each of the *dosha*s, but it is likely that one will dominate. If you are higher in one particular *dosha* then follow the dietary, seasonal, and lifestyle advice for that constitutional type. These are outlined in detail throughout the book.

If you have two *dosha*s with an equal or similar count then you have a mixed-*dosha* constitution and should do the following:

❀ For *vata-pitta*, follow a *vata*-reducing diet in the autumn and winter and a *pitta*-reducing diet in the spring and summer.
❀ For *pitta-kapha*, follow a *pitta*-reducing diet in the summer and fall and a *kapha*-reducing diet in winter and early spring.
❀ For *vata-kapha*, follow a *vata*-reducing diet in the summer and fall and a *kapha*-reducing diet in the winter and spring.

Whatever your overall constitution, you should choose the appropriate remedy for your current health imbalance.

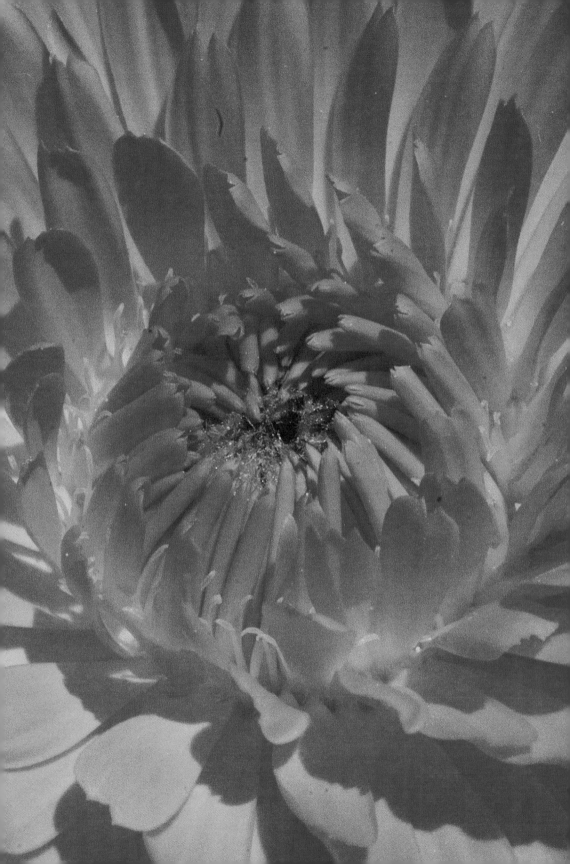

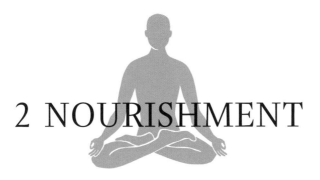

2 NOURISHMENT

> **"**The life of all living beings is based on food, and all the world seeks food. Complexion, clarity, good voice, long life, understanding, happiness, satisfaction, strength, and intelligence all come from food.**"**
> **CHARAKA SAMHITA**

There are two very important concepts in Ayurveda: *prana* and *agni*, the life force and the digestive fire. Ayurveda weaves myriad insights into how we can nurture these vital energies and make our lives full of health and wonder. So much of our existence centers on our appetite and digestion: how hungry we are, what we want to eat, how we feel before and after eating. Increasingly, we are reevaluating our food culture, its relationship to the environment, and how we are truly nourished. In fact, how we eat—in the broadest sense—is crucial to good health, and Ayurveda offers the tools for understanding why.

PRANA: THE LIFE FORCE

The food we eat brings us more than just nutrition and a sense of satisfaction—it brings us life. This vitality is the essence of food: its life force, known as *prana* in Ayurveda. Literally, *prana* is the "breath of life" that we absorb through breathing and by ingesting food. However, this depends on the vitality of the food you eat. Food that is filled with *pranic* life force is fresh, tasty, and healthy. It has absorbed the vitality of the soil it has grown out of, the water that has fed it, and the air and sun that it has grown in. Food high in *prana* is colorful, easy to digest, and easy to absorb. It is all you should eat if you want to be filled with life.

When our *prana* is healthy then our circulation is good and we are warm; our immunity is strong and we are protected; our breathing is easy and we are inspired; our muscles are strong and we are held; our energy is vibrant and we are animated; our appetite and digestion are good and we are nourished. *Prana* is not only beneficial, it is essential. For more on this concept, *see* Ecology, p.184.

The golden rules for healthy digestion

- Before you eat anything, make sure you are calm. If you are stressed, depressed, angry, or rushed it is better not to eat, or only very lightly.
- Don't eat while standing up or walking.
- Try and eat in a peaceful place—your food will taste better and digestion will be improved.
- Start each meal with something a little spicy to stimulate your digestion. Mix ¾-inch piece of freshly grated ginger, a squeeze of fresh lemon juice, and a pinch of salt to eat as a digestive chutney.
- Chew your food properly to ensure that your digestive enzymes get to work in the mouth and make it easier on the rest of your digestive system.
- Sip warm water with each meal but don't drink lots of fluids until at least an hour after finishing your food, as this can extinguish your digestive fire (*see* p.44).
- Don't eat incompatible foods (*see* box, p.63).
- Be aware of how your digestion is feeling before and throughout each meal. Follow your intuition and eat appropriately for your constitution (*see* p.64).
- "Stoke" your digestive fire with light, easy-to-burn, properly seasoned delights. Cook with digestive spices (*see* p.56).
- If you have any digestive troubles, it is best to eat until you are half-full of food and a quarter-full of liquid, leaving a quarter of your digestive capacity free for life-giving *prana* to circulate and help digestion.
- Eat your food with respect for nature and the gift of nutritious food she has bestowed upon you. Give thanks to the creator of your meal.

OUR FOOD CULTURE

"Even food, which is the life of living creatures, if taken in an improper manner destroys life."
CHARAKA SAMHITA

It hardly needs stating that we need food to live. Food gives us the bodily fuel that helps us grow, repair, metabolize, and energize. But it is also at the heart of how we, as a society, relate to ourselves and to nature. We seem to have a collective cultural "problem" with food that boils down to three main areas: how we eat, how we farm and what we eat.

Apart from giving us the nutrition we need, eating food is a simple way to feel emotionally "full," "complete," or "loved". If any of these things are lacking in our lives then we often turn to food as a support. I know I do. That is fine, as long as we have a healthy relationship with healthy foods most of the time. If we don't we are taking a one-way ticket to illness. So our first "issue" with food is how nourished we feel in ourselves. It is a huge question and one that we will look at again later (*see* Strength and Stillness, p.149).

Second, we take without giving back. Farmers traditionally understood, even without any knowledge of the complexities of soil chemistry, that in order to rear healthy plants you have to put organic matter back into the soil. Unfortunately, the agriculture industry's well-intentioned efforts to feed the world's growing population have focused on quantity and not quality. Agricultural inputs (fertilizers, pesticides, fungicides), heavily promoted and subsidised since the 1940s, give the possibility of increased production, but for a limited time only. Artificially stimulated growth disrupts the nutritional uptake of plants, leaving us with a diet that has an imbalance of nutrients. So our health, and that of the environment, is compromised.

Our third problem stems from what we eat. In the Western world we have an excess of poor-quality food, which is leaving people overweight yet undernourished. This condition is known as Type-B malnutrition. Type-A malnutrition occurs in a devastating famine, when there is literally no food to eat. Type-B is what happens when we have a sufficient or excess volume of food that is nutritionally bereft, resulting in a different type of devastation: chronic disease and premature aging.

Remarkably, only thirteen percent of men and fifteen percent of women in the more economically developed countries eat the recommended five daily portions of fruit and vegetables. Some authorities even suggest that we should be eating eight to ten portions of fruit and vegetables per day to provide adequate nutrition and antioxidant protection. Since 1950 our diet has consisted of 34 percent fewer vegetables, 46 percent more meat, 36 percent more fat (including harmful trans-fats), and 50 percent more sugar. Nearly 100 percent of the food we ate was organic back in the 1950s, whereas now this figure is less than three percent.

Our food is not only depleted by the excesses of intensive agriculture, but also by poor handling, processing, and storage practices. It doesn't take too much thought to work out that heavily processed foods aren't that good for you. In fact, during the last 50 years there has been a 50 percent reduction in food levels of vitamins A and C, omega-3 fats, iron, calcium, zinc, selenium, copper, and magnesium, as well as reductions in life-enhancing flavonoid and carotene content. What does this mean for our health? Let's look at just two minerals: magnesium and zinc. Magnesium is involved in over 300 essential enzyme reactions and zinc in over 100, and the health of virtually every major organ and system in the body depends in part on them. If our diet is deficient in these essential nutrients we will inevitably develop illnesses.

As if these problems were not enough, we are also faced with a toxic environmental onslaught that stresses our nutritional reserves even further. Unless people are extremely careful about what they eat, it is estimated that they consume 4 pounds 8 ounces of pesticides and 8 pounds 13 ounces of additives per year. Because most of these chemicals have only been present in the environment for a relatively short time, we have not yet been able to evolve a way to metabolize them. It is a huge challenge for our bodies, requiring even more nutrition to detoxify and eliminate these pollutants.

The body sustains and regenerates itself from the nutrition it receives. But if the food we eat is deficient in the vitamins, minerals, and micronutrients needed for our health, then we have a "nutritional gap." To ensure that our nutritional and health needs are met we really need to diversify our diet to include nature's finest healing roots, fruits, shoots, seeds, grains, beans, grass juices, vegetables, herbs, flower pollens, freshwater plants, seaweeds, and germinated sprouts. But when was the last time you ate all of these food families in one day? And if *you* didn't, who did?

FOOD AS MEDICINE AND FOOD AS POISON

"*There is nothing in the world which does not have therapeutic utility in appropriate conditions and situations.*"
CHARAKA SAMHITA

The connection between food, nutrition, and well-being is common knowledge. A healthy diet helps us to feel good and a poor-quality diet leads to illness. In fact, Ayurveda considers diet to be the most important factor in health and uses food for medicinal purposes as well as for nutritional effects. Herbal remedies, massage, exercise, and spiritual practice can balance and repair the body, but it is a "good" diet that gives us an easy, everyday opportunity to take control of our health.

Ayurveda has a theory that anything can be a food, a medicine, or a poison, depending on who is eating, what is eaten, and how much is eaten. We are all familiar with the phrase, "One man's food is another man's poison." For example, fresh gingerroot is a delicious flavor in food and helps digestion. It can be a stimulating medicine when used for therapeutic purposes, such as in a hot tea to ease a cold or induce a sweat. However, if too much is taken it can cause acidity and vomiting, hence acting as a poison in the wrong circumstances. That is why there is no strict Ayurvedic diet per se, only sage recommendations to help you find the tastiest and healthiest foods appropriate for your optimum health.

What is a food?

This seems like a pretty simple question but, looking at our food industry, real food is not always easy to find. A food is literally anything that you consume for nutritional purposes, whether it is of plant, animal, or mineral origin. You digest foods, plants, and herbs so that they become active in your body. Foods, just like herbal medicines, are complex substances made from a multitude of constituents, including fats, proteins, and carbohydrates, along with a host of phytonutrients (the natural components of plants that have health benefits without yet being determined as essential to life). These include flavonoids, carotenoids, alkaloids, and essential oils, and it is these nutrients which, when used appropriately, nourish and strengthen your body and facilitate its cleansing processes.

Let's take a look at what our modern food industry considers to be good food, using bread as an example. The "staff of life" was traditionally made from freshly ground wheat, natural leaven (wild yeast), water, with perhaps a little salt, and a few herbs for flavoring. But, oh, how far we've come from that recipe! The number of ingredients used today to make a loaf of bread is remarkable.

Modern industrial baking techniques require bread to be mixed with a range of "improvers" (e.g., E481 [sodium stearoyl-2-lactylate], E472e [mono- and diacetyl tartaric acid esters of mono- and diglycerides of fatty acids], E920 [L-cysteine], E282 [calcium propionate], and E202 [potassium sorbate]). E220 (sulfur dioxide), E300 (ascorbic acid), E260 (acetic acid), soy flour, vegetable fat, and dextrose are just some of the other things that you might find in commercially made bread. Your modern loaf could also contain flavoring and other "improver" ingredients, such as phospholipase, fungal alpha amylase, transglutaminase, xylanase, maltogenic amylase, hemicellulase, oxidase, peptidase (protease)—but, legally, the manufacturer wouldn't have to declare these on the label. Additionally, the bread is often made too quickly, creating carcinogenic acrylamides in the crust. Leavened with concentrated yeast (which may also include additives) in just a couple of hours, the bread is without many of the benefits of natural leaven.

For a proper health-giving fermentation, bread should leaven over an eight-hour period, using a natural sourdough process with a wild yeast "starter." This neutralizes phytic acid (which blocks calcium and iron absorption) and increases the bioavailability of nutrients such as vitamin B in the bran. Wild yeast contains gut-friendly lactobacillus bacteria (unlike candida-promoting concentrated industrial yeast), which assist with the assimilation of nutrients and the health of the digestive tract. Add this to a powerful digestive system and you get optimum absorption of high-quality food. In contrast, modern commercial bread often causes bloating and gas, and aggravates the nutritional state of the tissues and the microflora in the digestive tract. No wonder so many people are intolerant to it. This isn't what I call food.

What is a medicine?

The word "medicine" comes from the Latin *medico* ("I heal, cure"), itself derived from the Greek verb *medome* ("to take care of, think, execute with great art"). So, clearly, medicine is meant to be good for you. Intention and action, however, are often different and, although many products are labeled as medicines, it doesn't actually mean that they are.

Ideally, when we take a medicine, it is digested and transformed into a substance that prevents disease and heals the body. For example, when the common household spice turmeric is absorbed by the gut, compounds are released that encourage the body to produce a range of antioxidant and anti-inflammatory molecules. These give our innate inflammation response the necessary stimulus to help us heal; the spice acts to remove the symptom and the cause. What is more, turmeric, like most herbal medicines when used properly, has absolutely no negative side effects. I would call this a "true" medicine.

Contrast this with the average painkiller. When we swallow an aspirin, it is absorbed by the gut and inhibits the inflammatory response for the duration that its chemicals last in the body. Depending on the cause of the inflammation, its severity and the dosage, the aspirin may be sufficient to help the body recover from the inflammation. It is usually an effective painkiller. We all use it (about 120 billion tablets a year worldwide). But because it forces the body to do something, rather than encouraging its own defense systems, the drug will always have side effects. In aspirin's case these are usually minor, but in extreme cases it can cause internal bleeding, which in some people leads to death (over 1,500 each year in the UK). Although aspirin has been a temporary help, it has not removed the cause. This is why pharmaceutical drugs do not, in the absolute sense, heal the body and are therefore not "true" medicines because, by definition, they interfere with one process at the expense of another. It cannot be a cure if it causes another symptom.

What is a poison?

A poison is anything that causes damage or death to an organism, harming the cells, tissues and, organs in a body. It is antagonistic to health because it blocks, opposes, or reduces the natural functions of the body.

Accordingly, the painkiller described above would be a poison, as would most pharmaceutical chemicals. (For more on this subject, *see* Cleansing, p.79.) They can alleviate symptoms, but always have potentially harmful side effects because they block or reduce the natural vitality of the system. While I am not saying that all plants are medicines or that all pharmaceutical drugs are poisons, we do need to be mindful. Look at the information leaflet on any pharmaceutical drug and read about the long list of adverse reactions that may occur. What do you think— medicine or poison?

We know from Paracelsus, the great Renaissance alchemist, that the dose makes the poison. Or, as expressed by nineteenth-century English physician and educator Peter Mere Latham, "Poisons and medicines are oftentimes the same substances given with different intents." According to this definition, many so-called foods are poisons, too. Just consider the harmful cholesterol-raising and inflammatory effects of hydrogenated trans fats, or the blood-glucose swings caused by refined sugar that are implicated in diabetes.

This definition of a poison could be extended to anything that hinders the life force (*prana*) or the natural working of our body. Pharmaceuticals may be useful if a fever is raging out of control or if someone is bleeding heavily, but you need to be clear about exactly when, how often, and in whom these drugs are used. You may have to make the choice of using them one day.

YOUR DIGESTIVE SYSTEM

"It is obvious that that the body tissues cannot be nourished and developed when food is not properly digested by your digestive fire."
CHARAKA SAMHITA

Your digestion is at the center of your health. Ayurveda even goes so far as to say that poor digestion leads to every disease, and many insights can be gained from this. Ayurveda thinks of digestion as a fire, which is known as *agni* in Sanskrit. A warm fire burns well with good-quality, dry wood that is put on the fire at the right time in the proper place, with plenty of air to fan the flames. If you add a big wet log, it smokes and splutters; if you don't feed it enough, the fire goes out. And so with your own digestion.

Your digestive fire, or *agni*, is involved in many varied functions:
* having a regular appetite
* the taste of food
* digestion of food
* assimilation of nutrients
* absorption of both foods and experiences
* the experience of touch and feelings
* clarity of hearing
* your perception of the world
* feeling alert and awake
* clarity of thought
* feeling vital and energetic

When your *agni* is healthy it gives you your immunity, a sparkle in your eyes, and a warm luster to your whole body. A healthy digestive fire literally makes you glow. In terms of Ayurveda's more classical descriptions, *agni* is heating, lightening (it removes heaviness), sharp and penetrating, pungent (spicy) to taste and smell, and luminous and clear. Think of the sun. It is hot, burning, and transformative, just like *agni*. It is how you want your digestion to be. I often imagine the gentle flicker of a slow-burning and robust fire in the center of my belly and at the heart of all my cells.

When our digestive fire is balanced, it helps to make us feel positive, bringing confidence, happiness, optimism, enthusiasm, and a general feeling of being "on the ball." It gives us energy, vitality, passion, and the ability to find balance. We can meander through life's challenges and opportunities fairly happily when our digestion is good. When our digestion is out of balance, we are sluggish, muzzy-headed, stressed, and even a bit fearful, angry, and low. This low digestive strength also brings us poor energy and a feeling of being congested. It's as though our experience of life is "undigested" and is weighing us down. Notice how you feel after a big meal; probably tired, a bit bloated, and feeling heavy. This is because your *agni* is low. This isn't a problem once in a while, but if it is frequent then you need to do something about it.

If you know your particular type of digestive system (*see* box below) and how it reacts to the different challenges of your diet and your day, then you can understand how to keep your digestive fire working for you. It is the best way to perfect health. In fact, the simplest and most effective suggestion of any diet is to only eat when you are hungry. Your digestive fire will express its own innate wisdom and let you know when it is time to eat, when it is time to drink, and when it is time to rest. It really is that simple.

Learning to experience true hunger gives you an insight into the deeper workings of your self, your attachments to food, and how you are nurtured and cared for by what you eat. A beautiful way to love yourself is by giving yourself the food you really need. By all means treat yourself once in a while: a bit of organic dark chocolate tastes great and is wonderfully mood-enhancing. Just make sure that for the remaining 99 percent of the time you are giving yourself what you truly need to be healthy.

The four types of digestion

In Ayurveda there are four types of *agni* that categorize people's digestive tendencies. Can you recognize yours?

Balanced Regular hunger; food is well digested within 4 hours, with neither excess cravings nor lack of interest in food; bowels regular. These people feel great all the time.

Irregular Erratic appetite; frequent bloating; painful indigestion; intestinal cramps; constipation and dry stools; gurgling and gas. These signs are common in nervous *vata* types.

Intense Intense hunger but poor digestion; frequent loose stools and a burning sensation in the intestines; intense thirst and a parched mouth. These signs are common in fiery *pitta* types.

Weak Low appetite; slow digestion; heaviness after eating a meal; sluggish bowels and bulky stools; feeling cold; persistent sweet cravings and need for stimulants. These signs are common in sluggish *kapha* types.

UNDERSTANDING TASTE

The Sanskrit word for taste is *rasa*, and it is a very pregnant word: as well as taste, it can mean "essence," "juice," "sap," "lymphatic fluid," "flavor" and "delicious." Just saying the word sounds "juicy": *raa-ssa, rasa, RASA*. Flavor is the essence of life—it affects everything.

Remarkably, how we "taste" life affects our health and mood. It is probably my favorite "foodie" subject. Ayurveda identifies six tastes: sweet, sour, salty, pungent (spicy), bitter, and astringent, which we will discuss later. If your experience of life is "sweet" you are usually happy, while "bitter" episodes are less savory. Because our taste of life becomes our *rasa*, our essence, it is helpful to learn how taste affects us.

Imagine this: your bloodstream and cells are filled with the digested juices of what you eat, drink, and think. Whether a flavor is experienced as a sensation on your tongue or as an emotion in your mind, it produces the same physiological reaction. For example, your blood pressure can rise after you eat a spicy meal and also after an angry outburst. Hot spices, such as garlic, warm the mouth, stimulate metabolism, and raise the temperature of your whole system. This heat can also affect your consciousness and cause passionate moments or "hot-headed" behavior. Italians aren't famous lovers for nothing!

However, it is important to remember that a food's *rasa* is not static and can change depending on when it is harvested, where it is grown, how it is stored, and how it is processed or cooked. For example, immature fruits are more sour, whereas mature fruits are more sweet; garlic is very pungent when raw but becomes sweeter on cooking.

How you experience the "taste" of your life, be it on the physical, mental, or emotional level, depends on three of life's most important things: your digestive capacity, your constitutional tendencies, and your current state of health. That is why learning about taste is essential. Once you understand its effects, you can enter a whole new world of discovery about your life.

The effects of taste

Ayurveda states that every substance, including taste, has all of the five natural elements—Ether, Air, Fire, Water, and Earth—within it, but that usually only one or two are dominant. For example, the pungent flavor is dominated by Fire and Air and, like a fire and the wind, is hot, drying, and light. In addition to possessing elemental qualities, taste has a number of effects on the body and mind.

Temperature (hot or cold) Each specific taste affects the thermoregulatory and metabolic qualities in the body (i.e., heating it up or cooling it down). For example, cinnamon is pungent and hot, which raises body temperature; grapes are sweet and cooling, which can help to cool you down.

Quality (heavy or light, wet or dry, penetrating or soft) Taste also defines the qualities of whether a particular food is light or heavy to digest, and wet or dry on the mucous membranes. It also defines if the herb is penetrating or soft. For example, black pepper is spicy and also hot, light, dry, and penetrating: it is easy to digest, dries the mucus membranes, and penetrates deeply into the tissues. Chew on a peppercorn and these qualities will become clear.

Direction (where the food goes in the body) Tastes also have an affinity for certain parts of the body. We all know that garlic goes to our lungs as we can smell it on other people's breath. Asparagus is renowned for making our urine smell—Ayurveda knows asparagus is a bitter and cooling food that clears internal heat via the urinary system. Ginger has multiple "sites," clearing mucus from the lungs, warming the skin, invigorating the blood, and relaxing the muscles. Taste also has an effect on the movement of energy in the body, by influencing the direction in which *vata* (the *dosha* responsible for movement) travels. For example, the pungent taste (e.g., in chile) ascends and spreads energy outward, causing sweating, while the bitter taste (e.g., in coffee) descends, causing energy to move downward, sometimes with a laxative effect.

Dosha (effect on the constitution) Tastes also influence your *dosha*. For example, the sweet flavor builds earthy *kapha*, cools hot *pitta,* and reduces airy *vata*. As it is a nourishing taste, it increases the volume of all the tissues. Hence, it is no surprise that we live off sweet-tasting foods like wheat and rice, as they keep us strong.

A note on energetics

The science of energetics is the study of the transformation of energy. It is important to note that, when applied to food, energetics is not linear. For example, just because something is sweet does not mean that it will always increase moisture, weight, and *kapha*. It also depends on the other qualities in the substance: for example, whether it is dry or heavy or spicy. Nature is complex and manifests in similarly complex patterns and proportions. So, even though barley is sweet in taste, it is also slightly drying and acts as a diuretic (encourages urination), helping to clear excess fluids.

The energetic properties of foods also depend on how you prepare and use them. When peppermint is taken as a hot drink it causes sweating, but when it is drunk as a cold tea it reduces irritation and inflammation of the digestive tract. Cooking with nourishing herbs and foods is all about understanding the nature of the ingredient so that you know how its different qualities will be transformed. *See also* chart, p.63.

THE SIX TASTES

Ayurveda identifies six tastes, each of which has a different effect on the body and influence on the *dosha*s. We'll first look at the "science" of taste from the Ayurvedic perspective and later at a range of individual foods.

Sweet

Sweet is the flavor of strength and energy. It is associated with the elements of Earth and Water and is wet, heavy, and cool in quality. Foods or herbs with the sweet flavor, such as honey, rice, and oats, are considered to be tonics: they build and nourish all the tissues. Remember, we are talking about primary foodstuffs that are naturally sweet, not foods made from refined sugar. The sweet flavor from healthy foods increases your vital essence and the integrity of the immune system; the sweet flavor from refined sugars reduces them.

Sweet comes from sugars: glucose, sucrose, fructose, maltose, and lactose, which are made up of short (mono) and long (poly) chains of saccharides. Most foods, including many carbohydrates, fats, and proteins, are sweet.

The sweet flavor also has a mood: it is the flavor of love, sharing and compassion. We give candies to friends as gifts. It is also used to increase clarity and awareness of the spiritual aspect of life.

Sweet substances and experiences are moistening, so they increase the volume of wet *kapha*, cool hot *pitta,* and moisten dry *vata.*

The sweet taste also:
- heals tissue (e.g., aloe vera or licorice are often used for hastening wound repair)
- benefits and lubricates the mucus membranes lining the mouth, lungs, digestive, urinary, and reproductive systems
- helps to clear a dry throat and lungs by enhancing expectoration
- helps to remove the intense heat of *pitta* or "-itis" conditions (e.g., bronchitis, dermatitis)
- has a mild laxative effect and softens the stools
- is beneficial to skin
- improves hair and nail quality and is the best flavor for a making a smooth voice
- when digested properly, builds tissues, increases body mass, and creates strength

Following the great Ayurvedic principle of "like increases like," you generally want to increase your sweet experiences and flavors in life. However, in excess the sweet taste can reduce the strength of the digestive fire (*agni*), increase mucus production, create obesity, and promote congestion, so *kapha* types should exercise moderation. Too much sweetness can also cause toxins, fever, chest, and breathing problems, dampness, swollen lymph glands, flaccidity, heaviness, worms, fungal infections, intestinal dysbiosis, candida (thrush), obesity, and diabetes. It can also create cravings and greed. Exceptions to the rule of sweet substances increasing dampness are honey, mung beans, and barley: they are actually considered to balance excess moisture. You have to be on your toes with Ayurveda: there is always an exception to the rule!

Sour

The sour flavor is associated with Fire, together with a little Earth and Water, and creates both moisture and heat within us. Examples of sour foods are lemons, limes, and vinegar. The sour taste stimulates our digestion through its hot and light qualities and clears dryness with its capacity to promote fluids. Try sucking on a lemon: it immediately increases the flow of saliva. But if too much is eaten it draws the tissues inward and "puckers" the lips, making you shudder. This physical contraction can create an emotional reluctance to share things. Eating too much sour-tasting food encourages envy, and can make you feel like "sour grapes."

Sour is found in acids: citric, lactic, malic, oxalic, and ascorbic. These have a direct effect on digestion by promoting digestive secretions, especially via a reflexive action in the liver. This increases the flow of bile, which encourages the digestion of fats. Sour fruits such as lemons and amla (*see* The Pukka Pantry) are high in bioflavonoids (yellow pigment), which help absorb vitamin C and are considered to be antioxidant and rejuvenating. Most fermented foods are sour: cultured yogurt, sourdough breads, vinegar, pickles and alcohol. A little bit of these foods encourages digestion, but too much, especially of alcohol, can increase heat and mucus in the body.

The warmth and moisture of the sour flavor are good for dry *vata* types, but is not usually beneficial in hot and damp conditions.

The sour taste also:
❁ nourishes all the tissues, except the deepest reproductive tissue (it is believed to destroy semen and reduce fertility in both men and women)
❁ alleviates anxious *vata* disturbances of the nervous system, drawing scattered energy back in
❁ is a specific carminative, useful for digestion as it prevents the formation of gas

Use sour in moderation, especially if you are *kapha* or *pitta*, as it aggravates *pitta* heat and liquefies *kapha* wetness. In excess, it imbalances the chemistry of the blood and can cause dizziness, thirst, burning sensations, hyperacidity, ulcers, fever, itching, anemia, and skin diseases. It can also aggravate diarrhea, edema, and wet coughs and is not recommended in excessive congestive conditions. Amla, lemons, limes, and pomegranate seeds are the exception to the rule that the sour flavor aggravates *pitta*, as they actually reduce heat and inflammation.

Salty

The salty taste creates moisture and heat, and is wet, heavy, and hot. Try putting a grain of salt onto your tongue: it is instantly moistening; and a little sprinkle on food can kindle your digestive fire (*agni*). Its association with the Water element makes it a mild laxative and, with the Fire element, a digestive stimulant with antispasmodic properties.

Salty is an easily recognizable flavor. It has a sinking and heavy effect (rather like when you put some salt in a glass of water) that is very grounding for the nervous system. This is why the salty flavor is said to encourage stability. After all, we call people who are solid and reliable "the salt of the earth."

Salt is found in minerals and Ayurveda classifies different types: rock, sea, black, pink, and lake salt. Rock salt is considered the best as it is high in minerals and has fewer negative effects (*see* below). Salty is the flavor most rarely found in food, but seaweeds and celery are good sources.

The use of salt is a good lesson in the importance of dosage. Taken in correct quantities, salt is vital to our existence and is as essential to our health as water and food. It can save life when there is dehydration. But, in contrast, too much will cause ulcers and aggravate stomach acidity. Excess salt consumption also causes water retention, with resultant edema and high blood pressure. This physical "holding" is reflected in its emotional effects, as it is thought to lead to greed and dissatisfaction. So, even though it brings flavor to food, it encourages the desire for more flavor, more taste.

Salt reduces dry *vata*, as it creates both moisture and heat.

The salty taste also:
* stimulates the appetite, moistens dryness, and nourishes the nervous system
* is both a mild laxative and an emetic (induces vomiting) at the appropriate dosage (always be guided by a qualified practitioner)
* when used externally as a "salt pack" (wrapped in a cloth), it has warm and light qualities that reduce *kapha*, draw moisture out of the body, and heal wounds (only to be performed by a qualified practitioner)
* softens lumps and tumors

Salt aggravates hot *pitta* and wet *kapha*. In excess, it disrupts the composition of the blood and causes thirst, eye damage, ulcers, skin diseases, water retention, intestinal inflammation, hypertension, bleeding, gray hair, and baldness. Rock salt is the exception to the rule that salt is heating, as it has a cooling action and hence is used to rebalance high *pitta*. It also causes less water retention and damage to the eyes than the other types of salt.

Pungent (spicy)

The qualities of the pungent flavor are hot, dry, and light, as well as being penetrating and ascending. As such, it is associated with the elements of Fire and Air. Pungent foods and herbs, such as ginger, black pepper, and chile, are spicy. I am sure that you are familiar with the acrid heat of hot foods and spices spreading throughout your whole system, stimulating metabolism and helping digestion. On the mental level, too much heat, whether climatic or dietary, is known to cause "hot" emotions, ranging from passion and excitement to anger and irritation.

The pungent flavor is primarily found in essential oils, resins, oleoresins (such as myrrh), and mustard glycosides (found in brassicas), which are all used to stimulate, invigorate, penetrate, dry, and clear the accumulation of wet, stagnant, and congestive conditions. For example, the essential oils of ginger and black pepper are often used for clearing mucous congestion or warming a "cold" condition such as hypothyroidism. Pungent resins, such as guggul (Indian myrrh) and frankincense, are good detoxifiers, as they encourage vasodilation and the opening of the pores of the skin, enabling the body to sweat out unmetabolized toxins. Spicy teas literally "cook" any toxins that have accumulated.

The pungent taste works through irritation of local tissue and nerve endings. Food that is too spicy is painful. I will always be grateful to the man in India who, on seeing me suffering in the middle of eating a volcanic curry, gave me a spoonful of sugar. It was sweet relief.

Pungent foods are a panacea for wet *kapha*, drying the excess moisture and mucus prevalent in this constitution, season, and climate. It is also good for *vata*, but too much is drying and overly stimulating and this can aggravate scatty *vata*. The pungent taste also:

* benefits lung problems such as asthma or coughs where there is a buildup of mucus and congestion
* helps weight loss, as it reduces cholesterol and stimulates the metabolism
* removes cold, tense stiffness
* encourages the elimination of wind and digestive cramps

The heat of pungent herbs irritates *pitta* and should not usually be used where there is inflammation (exceptions to this are cardamom, cloves, coriander, cumin, and fennel). Ginger and cooked garlic are the exceptions to the rule that too much pungent flavor aggravates *vata*: in fact, they are beneficial, as they increase digestion and reduce intestinal gases. The pungent taste's drying effect on bodily fluids can reduce fertility and cause constipation. In excess, it creates burning, intestinal inflammation, bleeding, dizziness, thirst, urinary retention, lack of semen, reproductive disorders, and excessive dryness.

Bitter

The bitter taste is truly fascinating and one grossly underused in our diet. Relating to Air and Ether, it is dry, light, and cold. It creates space in the body by draining and drying excess fluids and is the ultimate detoxifier: by improving the function of the kidneys, liver, lung, skin, bowels, and lymphatic system, the bitter flavor helps toxins to be eradicated more effectively. Many bitter herbs have traditionally been considered to alter the chemistry of the blood and hence have been called "alteratives" or "blood purifiers." So, the bitter flavor helps to change our metabolism so that our absorption, assimilation, and elimination are improved.

However, too many bitter-tasting things encourage fear and anxiety and can actually "space you out," leaving you disorientated. Just remember the last time you had too much coffee. Many so-called "psychedelic" drugs and psychotropic plants (e.g., "magic mushrooms") are also bitter in taste. But it is the "lightening" quality of bitter that gives you access to the more subtle realms of consciousness. Lavender is a beautiful bitter, relieving anxiety and promoting good sleep.

The bitter flavor is often associated with a plant's defense mechanism and so many poisonous plants have a bitter taste. It is a simple evolutionary principle: taste nasty and no one will eat you! The bitter taste receptors are at the back of the tongue and are our last defense against poisoning ourselves. But not all bitters are poisonous. Commonly eaten bitter foods are coffee, asparagus, some salad greens like endive, and roasted chicory roots. Plants with bitter properties are known for their anti-inflammatory, antibacterial, fever-cooling, and digestive activities. Neem and andrographis (*see* The Pukka Pantry) are two well-known Ayurvedic bitters, famed for their ability to clear infection, heal skin problems, and purify the blood.

Bitter herbs are drying, cooling, and draining, and clear wet *kapha* and hot *pitta*. When treating *kapha* problems, bitter herbs are often combined with pungent ones to offset their cooling nature.

The bitter taste also:
* promotes bowel motions and urination
* helps with lung conditions, especially with infections manifesting in green and sticky mucus
* excels at clearing itching, swelling, and oozing skin
* stimulates the appetite and clears the palate, as well as encouraging the release of digestive enzymes (aperitifs are often a little bitter)
* kills worms and parasites in the intestines and blood (when used in high doses)
* soothes inflammatory *pitta* conditions of the skin, blood, and liver, such as hepatitis and jaundice
* is indispensable for treating heat in the intestines when there is dysentery, bleeding, and mucus
* benefits overweight conditions as it can dry and "scrape away" fatty accumulations

When misused or incorrectly prescribed, the bitter flavor can cause too much dryness and wasting, thereby aggravating dry *vata*. This can upset the nervous system and weaken the kidneys, causing constipation, excess urination, dizziness, reduction in semen, poor fertility, and dryness, coldness, and weakness of the whole body. Here's the exception: guduchi is a bitter herb that, along with the benefits given by its bitter flavor, is also an aphrodisiac and reproductive tonic due to its sweetness.

Astringent

Astringent is the driest flavor and holds things in place. Associated with Earth and Air, it is heavy, cold, and dry. As it draws inward it dries and reduces: when you eat something astringent your whole mouth contracts, drawing the mucus membranes closer together. Having too many "dry" and unfulfilling experiences can leave you with a lack of taste for life and even resentful at its lack of zest.

The astringent flavor is found in tannins. These polyphenols are particularly concentrated in the bark and leaves of trees and the outer rind of fruits. They are especially soluble in water; hence, the astringent taste and drying nature of a strong cup of black or green tea that is left to steep for too long. Astringency is often found in combination with plants that also taste sweet and/or sour.

Astringent clears damp *kapha* and hot *pitta*.

The astringent taste also
* holds tissues together and neutralizes bacteria (astringent herbs are often used as a wash to help heal wounds)
* helps to stop leakage of body fluids: bleeding (external and internal), excessive sweating, urination, diarrhea, excess catarrh, vaginal discharge, and premature ejaculation
* prevents loose and flaccid tissue from accumulating and can help with weight loss
* helps treat "sinking" problems, such as prolapses
* draws swelling inward, cools the heat of inflammations, and dries any damp suppuration

The astringent taste is usually detrimental to *vata* as it is too drying. Its cold and heavy quality can impair digestion and reduce the strength of the digestive fire. In excess, astringent flavors can cause *vata* conditions like rigidity, pain in the heart, convulsions, constipation, and gas. The haritaki fruit is a notable exception: because of its warming energy and sweet effect after digestion, it is one of Ayurveda's primary *vata* tonics, and forms part of its foremost formula, triphala (*see* The Pukka Pantry). In fact, Lord Buddha, in his manifestation as the Medicine Buddha, is depicted holding a haritaki fruit. That's how important an astringent fruit it is.

INGREDIENTS

Most important of all in a healthy diet is the food you prepare. Ensuring you get the best nutrition means that you should start with the best ingredients. This means fresh, unprocessed, and organically grown. In Ayurveda there are some essentials that should be in every pantry, and a number that, depending on your individual constitution, should be limited. For more on individual ingredients and their properties, *see* The Pukka Pantry.

 ## Grains

Grains, such as wheat, rice, barley, corn, millet, oats, are our basic staples. Whole grains, which contain all three parts (bran, germ, and endosperm), are healthier than the refined version—most of the nutrients are in the germ and the bran. One seed can grow hundreds of ripe kernels and it is this prolific energy that helps to create thoroughly nourished tissues. Grains are complex carbohydrates that release energy-giving sugars into our system in a regular and consistent fashion. They help to create balance in our lives and should make up the bulk of our diet. Grains are traditionally soaked and fermented for two to eight hours before eating to reduce nutrient-binding phytic acid and increase nutrient absorption and digestibility.

 ## Beans

Beans, such as lentils, kidney beans, and chickpeas, are excellent sources of protein. Their energetic quality is predominately drying. To ensure complete digestion they must be prepared properly by soaking for twelve hours and changing the water at least once. The best way to offset the dry, hard, and infamously gaseous qualities of beans is by cooking with moistening seaweeds, warming spices (asafetida, ginger, cumin), softening salts, and demulcent oils. Sprouted beans, which you can create yourself by placing soaked beans in a tray or cheesecloth bag for a few days, have high levels of enzymes and vitamin C and are useful cleansing foods.

 ## Vegetables

From roots to salad greens, vegetables offer wide-ranging benefits that are essential to the healthy diet of every constitutional type (*dosha*). Raw vegetables generally aggravate *vata*, as they are hard, cold, and difficult to digest, so Ayurveda recommends that everyone should eat vegetables when they are cooked and warm.

Fruits

In general sweet fruits, such as ripe grapes and blueberries, reduce *vata* and *pitta* but increase *kapha*. Sour fruits, such as cranberries, reduce *vata* but increase *pitta* and *kapha*. Dried fruits, such as figs, raisins, and apricots, all increase *vata* and should be soaked prior to use. If fruits are eaten at the same time as other foods, their digestion can be slowed, causing fermentation, gas, and bloating. Leaving a two-hour interval between eating fruit and other foods avoids this problem.

 Nuts and seeds

Salted and fried nuts and seeds aggravate all three *dosha*s, and any type of nut should be avoided by those with a sluggish, damp, and toxic *ama* condition (*see* Cleansing, p.72). If digestion is good they can be superb tonics to remove deficiency and build strength. Use fresh nuts and seeds where possible or freeze for long-term storage to protect their unstable oils.

 Meat and fish

All meat is heavy (with the exception of chicken), hard to digest, and best reserved as a nourishing tonic. If you eat meat it should be of the highest quality and eaten in small amounts. See p.60 for more details.

Sweet to taste, heavy and oily in quality, fish are strengthening and aphrodisiac. Fish reduces *vata* but increases *pitta* and *kapha*. Though oily fish are often proclaimed a beneficial source of essential fatty acids (omega-3 and -6), the pollution levels of the seas and their detrimental effect on the blood means that their health benefits may be mitigated.

> **The best Ayurvedic foods**
> Generally speaking, Ayurveda considers the most beneficial foods to be rice, wheat, barley, mung beans, asparagus, grapes, pomegranates, ginger, ghee (clarified butter), unpasteurized milk, and honey. These are all thought to be rejuvenating tonics to the tissues and digestion (provided the food is good quality and there are no intolerances). Ayurveda also recommends avoiding habitual use of "heavy" meats (e.g., beef), cheeses, yogurt, refined salt, processed foods, refined sugar, yeast, coffee, tomatoes, bananas, citrus fruits, and black lentils. These can create stagnation and undigested toxins, considered to be the scourge of health.

 Dairy

Dairy products, such as butter, yogurt, cream, ice cream, and ghee (clarified butter), hold a special place in Ayurveda. Because Ayurveda developed in India, where the cow is worshipped as a sacred animal, high-quality and properly prepared dairy products have a revered status and are central to its practice. The increasing intolerance to dairy appears to be caused by a combination of factors, principally pasteurization and homogenization, which destroy certain enzymes, making it more difficult to digest. Intolerance is also exacerbated by our own low digestive fire (*agni*) and excessive antibiotic use in livestock. These drugs enter the food chain, causing antibiotic resistance and disrupting digestion, so make sure your milk and dairy products are whole, organic, nonpasteurized, and non UHT. The mucus-producing properties of dairy products can be offset by using spices such as cardamom, black pepper, and ginger.

 Oils

The healthiest oils are sesame, olive, hemp, and virgin coconut (for ghee *see* Dairy). Oils should come from cold-pressed organic sources, and be stored in dark glass bottles at low temperatures. Those in clear plastic bottles can oxidize and go rancid, leading to inflammatory problems. The excessive use of oxidized or poor-quality hydrogenated oils (e.g., margarines) is one of the leading causes of diet-based disease. In *kapha*-aggravated conditions oils should be used in small quantities.

Herbs and spices

Herbs and spices not only bring flavor and aroma to food, they also help it become more digestible. Learning to cook made me realize how they can alter the way you feel—a Pukka meal isn't really "pukka" without them. Spices have mostly pungent, hot, dry, light, and digestive qualities, which largely come from the essential oils they contain. They reduce nervous *vata* anxiety and sluggish *kapha* stagnation, and increase *pitta* heat, stop spasms, ease gas, reduce mucus, remove heaviness, and can increase metabolism. Most also have potent antioxidant action. The best herbs and spices according to Ayurveda are basil, cardamom, cinnamon, coriander, cumin, fennel seed, ginger (fresh), mint, saffron, and turmeric. This is because, when used moderately, they balance all three *dosha*s, assist digestion and the absorption of nutrients, relax the intestines, clear wind, help *vata* descend and reduce the buildup of toxins. Importantly, they do this without being excessively hot or unbalancing to digestion. These ingredients should be your greatest friends in the kitchen.

What are herbs and spices?

"Herbs and spices" is the general term for ingredients that are used in the kitchen to provide flavor and digestive qualities. "Herb" normally describes leafy green seasonings with a gentle flavor, such as basil, cilantro, fennel leaf, oregano, parsley, rosemary, savory, and thyme. "Spice" normally refers to ingredients (usually from Asia) that are pungent and aromatic, such as black pepper, cardamom, chili, cinnamon, cloves, coriander seed, cumin, fennel seed, fenugreek, ginger, and turmeric.

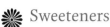 Sweeteners

All natural sweeteners, such as barley malt, date sugar, fructose, maple syrup, and rice syrup, are sweet and cooling, reducing *vata* and *pitta* but increasing *kapha*. Honey is sweet and slightly warming, while jaggery and molasses are excellent heating and strengthening tonics. Refined sugar should be avoided.

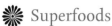 Superfoods

Superfoods have earned their special status because of the concentrated amounts of health-enhancing phytonutrients, vitamins, and minerals they contain. They usually offer some form of antioxidant and immune protection, resulting in us staying in better health. Some of my favorites are acerola berries, almonds, asparagus, blueberries, broccoli sprouts, chlorella, and spirulina.

 Water

Ayurvedic texts mention different types of water, each with different qualities: rain, spring, river, and well water, with rainwater being the most beneficial. It is now inadvisable to drink rainwater, so aim for purified water that does not contain chlorine, fluoride, and other chemicals. This is best achieved by using a water filter, as commercially bottled water has limited nutritional benefits.

Ayurveda is also very specific about drinking water at room temperature or even higher. Hot water is considered to be one of Ayurveda's best medicines: it kindles the digestive fire (*agni*), removes toxins, and refreshes the whole system. Chilled or iced water is inappropriate unless the weather is very hot. Try to avoid drinking too much after a meal as this can dilute your digestive juices and slow digestion.

Follow your thirst—do not just drink eight cups a day because you have read that you should, as this can lead to a weakened digestive fire and water retention. *Vata* types are prone to dryness, so they should drink the most; as *pitta* types are hot, they also need to drink quite large volumes of water; *kapha* types need the least amount of water, as they are already high in the water element.

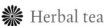 Herbal tea

Herbal teas are an excellent way to bring more liquids together with the health benefits of plants into your life. Herbal teas have many plus points: not only are they usually delicious, but as a warm drink they nurture digestion, encourage your circulation, and many can also soothe the nervous system. Most of the plants used for herbal teas are high in antioxidant molecules, and so one cup of herbal tea has the equivalent life-enhancing benefit of half a portion of fruit or vegetables.

THE VEGETARIAN CHOICE

I love being vegetarian. It tastes good, makes me feel good, and helps me feel part of a caring world. It's in my blood: my grandparents were pacifist vegetarian Quakers. When asked why am I vegetarian I say, "For every reason that there is to be." For me, these are environmental, economic, moral, health, spiritual and (now I know how to cook) because it is so utterly delicious. I am not saying it is necessarily the right choice for everyone—although perhaps I secretly believe it is.

Environmental and economic considerations

Vegetarianism is more environmentally sustainable. It is as simple as that. It takes 15 pounds 7 ounces of grain to produce 2 pounds 4 ounces of red meat and 4 pounds 8 ounces to produce 2 pounds 4 ounces of poultry. One-quarter of the earth's surface is now pastureland to support livestock. Three-quarters of all arable production in the US is destined for animal feed—grains and beans that could feed 800 million people. The livestock industry (meat, dairy, poultry, fisheries) uses 50 percent of all US water resources, with 13,198 quarts of water required to produce 2 pounds 4 ounces of red meat. The livestock industry is one of the largest contributors to environmental damage, creating seventeen percent of greenhouse gases (with transportation making up thirteen and a half percent of that figure). It is estimated that 50 percent of the world's rainforests have been cleared to support livestock for the meat industry, and 70 percent of the world's fish populations are threatened by overfishing. Enough said?

These figures show that it takes ten times as many resources to get our nutrition from meat as it does from grains. While it is not an absolute answer to the earth's environmental problems (because modern farming techniques as a whole need to be addressed), becoming a vegetarian is THE single most positive impact that an individual can have on the environment.

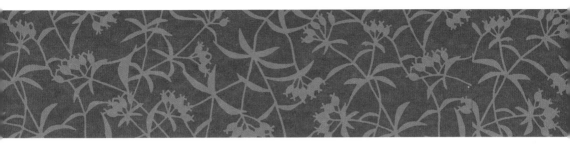

The moral choice

I don't think that being a vegetarian makes you an "absolutely" better or more moral person, but I do think it makes you relatively better. I mean, why would we kill another animal when we can get plenty of nutrition from plants? Of course, you may think we are superior to other animals or that we are naturally designed to be carnivorous. But why would we impose such fear and pain on another animal if we don't have to? If you have ever visited a battery chicken farm or seen cattle slaughtered at an abattoir you will know what I mean. However hard they try, all meat-eaters end up eating this sort of mass-processed meat because it is what is generally available in stores and restaurants.

The very nature of our existence means that we kill all the time: washing our hands destroys millions of bacteria; driving a car kills lots of insects; digging the earth kills lots of worms. So to live we must kill. But we do not necessarily have to eat another being. Fortunately, I have a choice not to eat meat—I don't live in the Kalahari Desert and "need" animal flesh to support me. I live in the UK, where vegetarian options are plentiful.

My intention is this: to try to live a life that causes no other beings intentional pain. This is the yogic attitude known as *ahimsa*, or nonviolence. It is the code of conduct that the Buddha recommended and the value that Gandhi lived by. Being vegetarian doesn't make you peaceful—ask my calm but chicken-loving wife about my occasional lapses of sense of humor. But it is a way of identifying your intention: vegetarianism induces a moral code by which I can attempt to live.

The case for health

The health reasons to be vegetarian are legion. Generally speaking, vegetarians suffer less from heart disease, diabetes, cancer (breast, bowel, prostate, pancreatic), hypertension, gall-bladder problems, obesity, and osteoporosis than nonvegetarians. Vegetarians also make fewer visits to their doctor and spend less time in hospital (about 22 percent less than a meat-eater). It sounds like a good opportunity for a vegetarian tax break

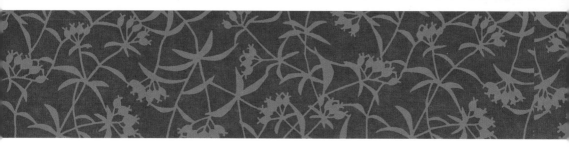

and a reduced insurance premium to me. It is nevertheless all too easy to eat an unhealthy vegetarian diet of white bread, lots of cheese, and processed foods. You can also be a meat-eater while at the same time including high levels of vegetarian foods. Eating a healthy vegetarian diet means that you exceed the government-recommended levels of fruit, vegetable, whole grain, fiber, and low-saturated fat consumption. Vegetarian foods also contain high amounts of various "super-nutrients," such as protective antioxidants, healing phytochemicals, and essential micronutrients, known to protect from a host of degenerative diseases.

Ayurveda considers that foods have different qualities that affect the makeup of the body–mind. Ayurveda divides nature into three forces or qualities, known as *trigunas*: *sattva, rajas,* and *tamas* (*see* Strength and Stillness, p.138). *Sattva* refers to qualities of balance, equality, and stability. It is light and luminous and holds the capacity for happiness. *Rajas* generates activity, change, and disturbance. It is mobile and excitable, causing dispersion and disintegration. *Tamas* is the immobile, "stuck" quality. It is heavy and results in delusion and confusion. Generally speaking, vegetables, fruits, nuts, grains, and milk (organic) are considered to be *sattvic* and increase awareness; meat is considered to be *rajasic* and increases the passions; and processed foods are considered to be *tamasic* and induce low energy.

Of course, what is appropriate for each individual must be taken into account, but a well-balanced vegetarian diet can enhance the quality and length of your life.

When not to be vegetarian

There are a few times in life when there are some good reasons not to be vegetarian. Anyone who is undernourished or recovering from a debilitating illness is a candidate for a bit of chicken soup. New mothers and those continuing to breastfeed often need a bit of extra animal protein.

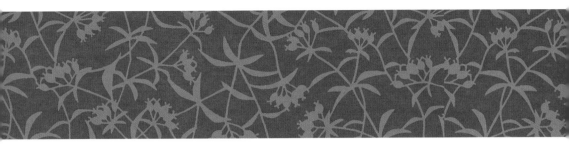

If you do eat meat, keep the portions to about 1$^1_4$ ounces a couple of times a week, and insist on organically sourced, grass-fed animals. Animals need to be free-range and grass-fed in order to access a range of plant nutrients. This gives the meat a healthy balance of essential fatty acids and higher levels of conjugated linoleic acid (CLA), which has immune-potentizing properties. Cook all meats with digestive spices (*see* p.56) to counteract their "heavy" quality and include lots of grains, beans and vegetables.

The Ayurvedic view of vegetarianism

Ayurveda is not a moralistic system, although morality does infuse its practices. As a science in pursuit of health, it is primarily but not wholly vegetarian. If someone's health can benefit from eating some animal meat, then this is recommended. Ayurveda would understand that there is some *karma*, or effect, from using animal products, but argues that the health of the individual is paramount. That said, it does recommend a primarily vegetarian diet which is easy to digest. Also in accordance with *karma*, it would encourage an awareness of one's actions and there is little doubt that the massive impact of today's meat industry on the environment, economy, and health of society would have influenced the opinion of the founding sages of Ayurveda.

Spiritual reasons to be vegetarian

At the very heart of being a vegetarian is its spiritual quality. Spiritual in the sense of connecting with the part of life that honors all beings as an expression of unconditional love. Spiritual in the sense of distancing oneself from the material world to a more contemplative place, where you can reflect on who you are and what you are doing here. Spiritual in distinction to material flesh. Before we get too purist about it, I am sure that many enlightened yogis have eaten meat; it's just that some of us need all the help we can get to live a spiritually enlightened life. If you want it to be so, vegetarianism can form part of your spiritual practice.

SEASONAL, LOCAL, AND ORGANIC

So many of our health imbalances are due to the climate we live in and the diet we eat. Eating a seasonal diet and as much locally grown food as possible can help us align with our environment. Indigenous or locally grown foods can offset the impact of the local climate: watermelons grow in desert regions, helping to "moisturize" the body against the harsh dryness of summer; refreshing salads are mainly in season when it is hot, helping to keep the body cool; in northern Europe an abundance of warming root vegetables help to "dry" the effects of wet winters.

It is now well documented that organic foods and herbs have higher levels of both primary nutrients and secondary metabolite compounds than conventionally grown crops. I am fascinated by these secondary plant metabolites: they give plants most of their therapeutic value, vibrant taste, and energetic qualities. This means the metabolites in organic crops are more potent and thus more effective.

A recently concluded EU-funded research program on Quality Low Input Food concluded that, "Levels of a range of nutritionally desirable compounds (e.g., antioxidants, vitamins, glycosinolates) were shown to be *higher* in organic crops." Conversely, "Levels of nutritionally undesirable compounds (e.g., mycotoxins, glycoalkaloids, cadmium, and nickel) were shown to be *lower* in organic crops." In addition, levels of fatty acids, such as gamma linolenic acid (GLA) and omega-3, were 10–60 percent higher, Vitamin E 50 percent higher, and beta-carotene was 75 percent higher in organic milk and dairy products, and levels of Vitamin C were up to 90 per cent higher in leafy vegetables and fruits.

Another benefit of using organic herbs and foods is that you reduce your exposure to potentially toxic pesticides. In 2006 the European Commission said, "Long-term exposure to pesticides can lead to serious disturbances to the immune system, sexual disorders, cancers, sterility, birth defects, damage to the nervous system, and genetic damage."

The Soil Association (the UK's leading organic charity) says, "Organic farming and food systems are holistic, and are produced to work with nature rather than to rely on oil-based inputs such as fertilizers. Consumers who purchase organic products are not just buying food which has not been covered in pesticides (the average apple may be sprayed up to sixteen times with as many as 30 different pesticides), they are supporting a system that has the highest welfare standards for animals, bans routine use of antibiotics and increases wildlife on farms."

Ayurveda supports living as natural a life as possible. Today this requires some flexibility, but by taking on board a few simple and natural practices you will see your health transformed on a very profound level. *See also* Ecology, p.176.

WHAT GOES WRONG WITH DIGESTION?

The digestion system is very complex and it is relatively easy for it to go out of balance. It faces an intense daily onslaught: over- or undereating; foods with imbalanced mineral ratios, a distorted fat balance, and high in refined sugars; antibiotics, anti-inflammatories, harsh laxatives, hormone treatments, and so on. In addition, eating too many preserved, stale, cold, or sticky foods results in something called "intestinal dysbiosis." We call this low digestive fire, or low *agni*, in Ayurveda. The digestive system becomes out of kilter, potentially leading to "leaky gut" syndrome, where larger than intended protein molecules pass into our bloodstream and cause multiple sensitivities. This results in the formation of poor-quality *prana* from the food, which leaves the body tissues poorly nourished. Following the advice in this chapter should avoid or solve any of these problems.

Food combining

As you have seen, different foods have different tastes and qualities, and building or cleansing effects. If foods with different energetic qualities (*see* box, p.47) are combined they can cause incompatibilities that upset digestion. This ultimately results in food intolerances and other health imbalances. Those foods listed in **bold** in the chart below are the most significant incompatibles.

A few substances act as antidotes to the negative effects of certain foods. For example, black pepper reduces mucus from dairy products and makes cucumber easier to digest; cardamom lessens the overstimulating, *vata*-aggravating effect of caffeine; ginger and black pepper make potatoes less "heavy" and easier to digest, while using ghee and olive oil makes them less dry and aggravating to *vata*.

Food type	Incompatible with	Exceptions
Fruit	**Other food.** All fruit should be eaten at least two hours away from other foods	Dates and milk
Milk	**Bananas**, bread, **eggs**, yogurt, fish, meat, melons, cherries, sour foods	
Yogurt	Fruit, **milk**, meat, *Solanaceae* family, eggs, fish	
Eggs	**Milk**, fruit, yogurt, cheese, fish, meat	
Grains	Fruit	
Beans	Fruit, cheese, eggs, yogurt, milk, fish, meat	
Lemon	Milk, yogurt, tomatoes, cucumbers	
Honey	Ghee in equal weight (1 teaspoon honey equals 3 teaspoons melted ghee)	Honey should not be heated, but adding honey to a warm drink is all right
Radishes	Bananas, raisins, milk	
Raw food	Cooked food	
Fresh food	Leftovers	

EATING RIGHT FOR YOU

"When diet is wrong, medicine is of no use.
When diet is correct, medicine is of no need."
AYURVEDIC PROVERB

For ultimate health, your diet can be tailored to your particular constitution. If you are a combination of *dosha*s, then look at the recommendations made in Constitution, *Pukka Practice*, p.30. However, if you are intolerant to any food or simply don't like it, then avoid it. In all cases, try to eat primarily vegetarian and organic (*see* previous pages).

Top tips for the healthy vegetarian

I have seen too many unhealthy vegetarians (and vegans) in my clinic. It is essential for vegetarians to eat an especially healthy diet. This takes a fair bit of effort—soaking, boiling, and kneading—but it can be fun and has results.

You MUST eat lots of whole grains, beans, and nuts. Include seaweeds and herbs and spices in your diet (ginger, turmeric, cumin, and coriander are essentials). One easy way to do this is to cook your rice and vegetables in deeply nourishing concentrated "stocks" that contain herbs, spices, and vegetables. Make sure you are getting the correct balance of healthy oils, particularly omega-3 and omega-6 (where the ratio should be 1:2). Vegetarian sources of omega-3 do not convert very well to docosahexaenoic acid (DHA) and eicosapentaenoic acid (EPA), so keep your levels of hemp and flaxseed high, while reducing your intake of omega-6 oils. Ayurveda recommends taking ghee with food (2 teaspoons per day) to nourish the tissues.

It is important to supplement your diet with superfoods and specialist "pukka" herbs (*see* The Pukka Pantry): use chywanaprash, the herbal tonic jam, and rejuvenating herbs such as ashwagandha, aloe vera juice, and ginseng when appropriate. For an extra nutritional boost add goji berries to oatmeal, put shatavari in rice pudding, and mix amla berries into soups. Because of difficulties in getting enough Vitamin B12, as well as the pervasive nutritional depletion in the food chain, I would recommend supplementing with a whole food multi-vitamin as well.

THE *VATA* DIET

This regime nourishes the nervous system, raises the digestive fire (*agni*), and aids the absorption of nutrients. Follow this diet if you are predominantly a *vata* type, or are suffering from a *vata* imbalance, as it is useful for relieving nervous tension, cramps, pain, anxiety, coldness, insomnia, bloating, constipation or pebble-like stools, and dryness. It is particularly valuable at the *vata* times of year, which are primarily spring and fall.

In general:
* eat at regular times
* eat to less than full
* practice relaxation
* emphasize foods that are warm, soupy, heavy, and oily
* favor foods that are sweet, sour, or salty
* reduce foods that are cold, dry, or hard
* reduce foods that are very spicy, bitter, or astringent
* avoid yeast, refined sugars, coffee, tea, tobacco, drugs, poor-quality oils, and extremely spicy foods
* supplement your diet with chywanaprash

Grains Rice (basmati, brown, wild), wheat, oats (cooked), and quinoa are very good. Amaranth is fine in moderation, but reduce barley, corn, millet, buckwheat, and rye, as these are a little drying and can be difficult to digest, creating wind.

Beans Avoid all beans, except for marinated tofu and mung beans and, occasionally, red lentils.

Vegetables Avocado, beet, cucumber, carrot, sweet potato, and seaweeds are the best. Peas, brassicas, and leafy green vegetables, summer and winter squashes and potatoes are best well-cooked in oil or ghee with mild, digestive spices. Avoid the *Solanaceae* (nightshade) family (unless potatoes are cooked as above). Raw vegetables, especially onions, should also be avoided, as these all create wind.

Fruits Favor sweet, sour, or heavy fruits, such as berries, banana, grapes, cherries, all citrus fruit, fresh fig, peach, melon, plum, fresh dates, pineapple, mango, and papaya. Cooked apple and pear are fine. Soaked prunes and raisins should be taken in moderation, but avoid dried fruits, uncooked apple and pear, pomegranate, and cranberries, as these can create wind.

Nuts and seeds All are good in moderation, especially when soaked.

Meat and fish Seafood and a little chicken and turkey are fine; beef should be avoided as it is difficult to digest.

Dairy All dairy products are nourishing, particularly yogurt. Always boil milk before you drink it, mix with cardamom seeds, and drink it warm. Don't take milk with a full meal or with fruit. If intolerant, substitute with almond or rice milk. Avoid ice cream, powdered milks, and soy milk. Cook with plenty of ghee to moisten "dry" foods.

Oils All oils reduce dryness and are nourishing. Emphasize hemp, sesame, olive, sunflower, and flax.

Herbs and spices All are fine, particularly asafetida, cardamom, cumin, cilantro, ginger, fennel, dill, cinnamon, salt, cloves, mustard seed, and black pepper. These help reduce gas and spasms in the digestive system.

Sweeteners All are good, especially honey, molasses, barley malt, and maple sugar. Avoid all refined white sugar.

Superfoods Asparagus and spirulina are particularly nourishing for *vata*.

Drinks Take plenty of warm water and spicy and relaxing herbal teas, such as ginger and chamomile.

THE *PITTA* DIET

This heat-reducing diet is useful for predominantly *pitta* types, or for those suffering from *pitta* imbalances, such as inflammations, skin conditions, itching, yellowing of the eyes, urine, and stools, loose and smelly stools, joint pain, hot flushes, acidity, ulcers, bitter taste in the mouth, anger, irritation, infections, and fever. It is particularly beneficial in late spring.

In general:
- ❀ include cooling aloe vera juice daily
- ❀ emphasize foods that are cool, refreshing, and liquid (e.g., fresh fruits and vegetables)
- ❀ favor foods that are sweet, bitter, or astringent
- ❀ reduce foods that are spicy, salty, or sour
- ❀ avoid pungent foods
- ❀ avoid alcohol, coffee, tea, yeast, chocolate, cheese, yogurt, and meat; also avoid low-quality oils, which increase inflammation

Grains Increase wheat, basmati rice, barley, and oats. Reduce corn, rye, millet, and brown rice.

Beans Tofu, mung beans, aduki beans, chickpeas, kidney beans, and lentils all reduce *pitta*. Avoid all others.

Vegetables Favor avocado, cucumber, cooked beet, sweet potato, leafy green vegetables, pumpkin, summer squash, broccoli, cauliflower, celery, ladies fingers, lettuce, sprouted beans, peas, green beans, and seaweeds. Keep potato, cooked spinach, and olives to a minimum, and avoid the rest of the *Solanaceae* (nightshade) family. Also avoid alliums, especially raw onions, garlic, and radishes, and raw beet, spinach, and mustard greens, as these all increase heat and acidity.

Fruits Favor sweet fruits such as grapes, lime, cherries, all types of melon, coconut, pomegranate, mango, apple, berries, fully ripened orange, pineapple, and plum. Reduce sour fruits such as grapefruit, lemon, papaya, unripe orange, pineapple, and plum.

Nuts and seeds Hazelnuts and sunflower seeds are good. Avoid peanuts, as these can create inflammation.

Meat and fish Chicken, pheasant, and turkey are preferable, but beef and seafood increase inflammation.

Dairy Milk, butter, and ghee are good for pacifying heat. Avoid sour and fermented foods like yogurt, cheese, sour cream, and cultured buttermilk. Also avoid egg yolk.

Oils Flax, hemp, borage, evening primrose, olive, sunflower, and coconut oils are best. Reduce sesame, almond, and corn oil.

Herbs and spices Cinnamon, coriander, dill, anise, cardamom, fennel, turmeric, fresh ginger, and small amounts of black pepper are good, but asafetida, ginger powder, cumin, fenugreek, clove, celery seed, salt, and mustard seed strongly increase heat and should be taken in moderation. Chili powder and cayenne should be avoided.

Sweeteners All natural sweeteners are good, except for honey and molasses.

Superfoods Aloe vera juice, asparagus, chlorella, spirulina, and wheatgrass juice all help to cool the system and clear inflammation. Almonds are also good.

Drinks Cool drinks, and minty and refreshing herbal teas.

THE *KAPHA* DIET

This regime reduces fluid and congestion and can be followed by predominantly *kapha* types, or those suffering from a *kapha* imbalance, such as sinus congestion, a thick tongue coating, paleness, high cholesterol, and edema (swelling). It is also useful for banishing tiredness, heaviness, and sluggishness and is particularly beneficial during the winter months.

In general:
* eat only when you are hungry and not between meals
* emphasize foods that are light, dry, or warm
* favor foods that are spicy, bitter or astringent
* include ginger in your daily diet: take a pinch of fresh gingerroot root with a few drops of lemon juice before each meal
* reduce foods that are heavy, oily, or "cold"
* reduce foods that are sweet, salty, or sour
* avoid overeating, especially at night
* do not eat raw or refrigerated foods
* avoid yeast, salt, cheese, yogurt, chocolate, refined sugars, flour, low-quality oils, and meat

Grains Increase barley, corn, buckwheat, quinoa, rye, and millet, as these are slightly drying and/or warming. Avoid or reduce intake of wheat and oats, as they increase heaviness and congestion. The sweet nature of rice is generally aggravating for *kapha*, although the lightness of basmati and wild rice make them acceptable.

Beans All beans are fine, except tofu, which is very cold and hard to digest.

Vegetables Increase eggplant, beet, broccoli, cabbage, carrot, cauliflower, celery, green leaves, kale, potato, pumpkin, alliums, Brussels sprouts, and seaweeds. Reduce avocado, ladies fingers, olives, tomato, cucumber, sweet potato, and summer squash, as these increase fluids.

Fruits Lighter fruits, such as apple and pear, are better, especially if baked or stewed. Reduce sweet, heavy, or sour fruits such as orange, banana, pineapple, fig, date, coconut, and all types of melon, as these increase heaviness and congestion.

Nuts and seeds In general, reduce nuts as they are too oily. Pumpkin and sunflower seeds are fine.

Meat and fish White meat from chicken or turkey is fine, as is seafood. Avoid or reduce red meat and pork, as they are too congesting.

Dairy Milk diluted with water is better, or use goat milk. Always boil milk first, preferably with cardamom or ginger to help reduce any mucus-generating properties, and drink it warm. Do not drink milk with a full meal, or with sour or salty food. A little ghee is fine. Avoid butter, eggs, cheese, yogurt, buttermilk, and buffalo milk.

Oils Reduce all oils. Virgin coconut oil is fine for frying. Use hemp, flax, and sunflower as cold-pressed oils straight onto food (i.e., not for cooking).

Herbs and spices Include all spices, especially ginger. Avoid salt, which increases water retention and mucus.

Sweeteners A little honey (2 teaspoons/day) helps to reduce congestion. Reduce all other sugar products.

Superfoods Aloe vera, almonds, asparagus, broccoli sprout and chlorella can help to cleanse the system.

Drinks Hot drinks and spicy and warming herbal teas, such as ginger, cinnamon, and fennel.

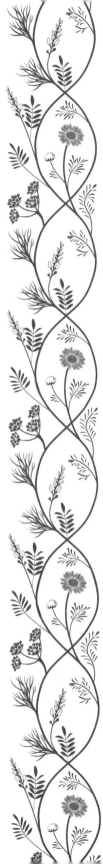

PUKKA PRACTICE

HOME TESTING FOR FOOD INTOLERANCES

My clinical experience has shown me that as many as 50 percent of us are intolerant to some degree to certain foods. A food intolerance is described as an immediate or delayed adverse reaction after eating a specific food. It is slightly different to a full-blown allergy, which is diagnosed through an immunoglobulin E (IgE) test and may indicate some propensity to anaphylaxis. There is some discrepancy between orthodox and holistic circles as to the exact definition, but both accept that an intolerance or allergy can be identified and—except in cases of severe anaphylactic allergies—your body trained to tolerate the food in question.

Sensitivity to foods usually forms slowly by repetitive and habitual eating of a certain food. A couple of centuries ago we used to eat over 200 different species per year, while today at least 80 percent of our diet comes from about twenty species. Our consumption of certain foods, particularly denatured ones like processed dairy, wheat, soy, and sugar, is so intensive that it is not surprising we can acquire an intolerance to them.

Food allergies and intolerances have been linked to a wide variety of diseases, affecting the following systems: gastrointestinal, genitourinary, immune, mental, emotional, musculoskeletal, skin, respiratory, membrane, and heart. Common signs and symptoms of intolerances are bloating, intestinal cramps, acid indigestion, poor digestion, chronic diarrhea, constipation, dark circles and puffiness under the eyes, inflammation of various types, headaches (including migraine), chronic runny nose, itchy eyes, asthma, hives, eczema, psoriasis, acne, mental and physical fatigue, inflammatory diseases (e.g., arthritis, Crohn's disease), and chronic infections.

Experimenting with the foods you eat can help you to tune in to your digestion. It is also the best way to discover food intolerances. You may want to experiment even if you don't display any typical symptoms, as food intolerances do not always manifest in the gut. Once any intolerance has been identified, the body can usually be reeducated into accepting the food by following the guidance below.

Testing for an intolerance

Select one common food at a time, starting with one that you eat the most, and completely remove the item from your diet for two full weeks. Read the labels of all the foods you eat to ensure that nothing creeps in. Make sure that you have helpful replacements for the food at hand so that you can more easily keep to your task (*see* the chart below). Then, after two weeks, eat a medium to large amount of the suspect food. The two-week abstinence period allows the body to mount a stronger response, making intolerance easier to identify.

If its reintroduction causes a noticeable negative reaction (e.g., one or more of the symptoms listed above) over the next 24–48 hours, you are probably intolerant to the food and should remove it from your diet for the time being. If there is no response, you are not intolerant to this food, and may consume it freely. If you are unsure of your response, you should retest.

Once you have identified the culprit, you should eliminate that food from your diet for three to six months. After a break of this length, many people find they can then start to eat the food occasionally (which means not more than once every four or five days) without a reaction occurring. Eating the food for several days in a row will probably reactivate the intolerance and cause a return of symptoms.

Although any food can create problems, the following are the ones that most commonly cause intolerance. Where appropriate, a substitute food has been recommended. Take care not to substitute with another known allergen.

Food	Suggested substitute	Food	Suggested substitute
Cows milk	Goat milk, rice milk, almond milk	Coffee	Herbal tea
		Tea	Herbal tea
Wheat	Wheat-free substitutes	Alcohol	Fruit juice
Corn	Other grains	Nuts	Other protein source
Chocolate	Carob	Oats	Quinoa
Egg	Egg-free substitutes	Yeast	Natural leaven (for making bread)
Refined sugar	Honey, molasses		
Orange	Other citrus fruits	Dried fruits	Nuts
Cheese	Goat cheese	Apple	Alternative fruit
Tomato	Beet	Peach	Alternative fruit
Potato	Sweet potato	Banana	Alternative fruit
Carrot	Parsnip, pumpkin	Strawberry	Alternative fruit
Rye	Other grains	Melon	Alternative fruit
Rice	Other grains	MSG (or E621)	Homecooked food; seaweed for salty flavoring
Fish	Other protein source		
Grapes	Pomegranates	Benzoic acid (food preservative)	Homecooked food
Onion	Asafetida		
Soya products	Hemp, rice, or almond milks	Beef	Other protein source
Pork	Chicken	Chicken	Other protein source
Peanut	Almonds		
Walnut	Almonds		

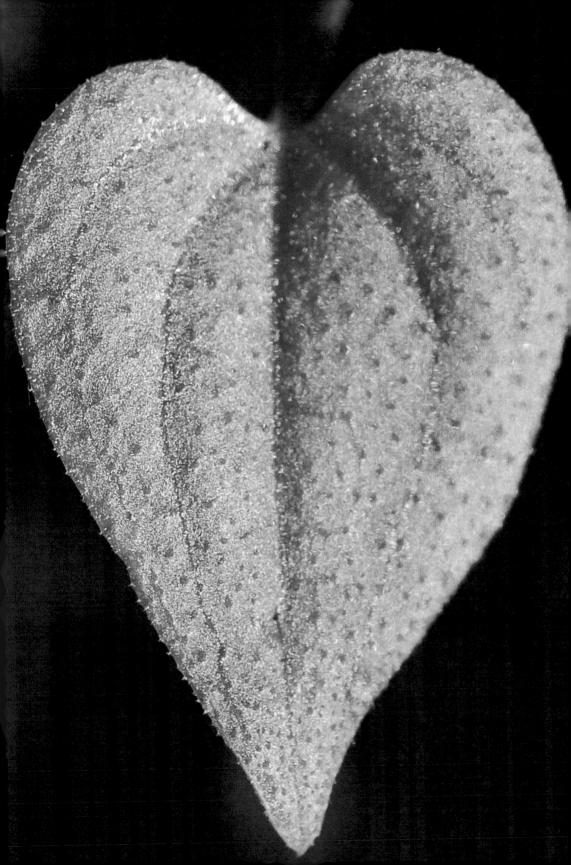

3 CLEANSING

> **"***When food is undigested because digestion is low it becomes imbalanced and collects in the stomach. It is known as *** ama.***"**
> ***ASHTANGA HRIDAYA SAMHITA***

We are all familiar with feeling under par, usually after we've been overdoing it: eating too much, drinking too much, doing too much. In addition, our systems can become "clogged up" with environmental pollutants and media overload. When this occurs we need to cleanse and refresh ourselves to feel balanced. We wash our hands and face every day and this helps us to feel revitalized: think how renewed you feel after a warm bath. Just as our skin needs regular cleansing, so do our insides. If we don't, toxins accumulate—known in Ayurveda as *ama*—and we get ill. The body routinely rids itself of waste matter: we normally urinate, excrete, and sweat daily. But because we cannot scrub our inner body we need to learn a few skills to help cleanse our tissues, organs, and mind. This is the art of Ayurveda.

THE CONCEPT OF *AMA*

Central to the Ayurvedic view of cleansing is its unique concept of *ama*. It has no direct equivalent in modern medicine but can be loosely thought of as toxic material. Literally, the Sanskrit word *ama* means "unripe, uncooked, immature and undigested." According to Ayurveda, a toxin is an unmetabolized substance not used by your body or assimilated by your mind. It can be created from foods or experiences that are absorbed but then not used, or from ones that remain undigested, creating fermentation and imbalance in all three *doshas*. I think of a toxin as anything that does not serve my life anymore, but is still "hanging around." It may be yesterday's poorly digested supper, last week's argument, last year's shock, or last decade's disappointment.

Ama, or toxic material, is the bed in which disease flourishes. Toxins have damp, sticky, heavy, and stagnant qualities. They cause "stuckness" and stagnation. They prevent change, growth, and evolution. Toxins can mingle with heat, causing inflammation and infection. They can accumulate with cold, leading to growths and blockages. They can irritate the nervous system, leading to clouded thinking. Just think of that "heavy" feeling that persisted after you last had a cold. Remember the last time you were depressed and felt "stuck in the mud." That is *ama*.

Modern medical terms for the signs of *ama*

It is always difficult to translate traditional terminology and concepts directly into today's medical language. However, some of the problems associated with systemic toxicity include:

- high cholesterol; high triglycerides; atherosclerosis; heart disease
- high blood-sugar levels; late-onset diabetes
- rheumatoid conditions; arthritis; gout
- bacterial, viral, and fungal infections; excessive candida in the mouth/gut/vagina
- high levels of free radicals; oxidative damage
- some forms of depression; dementia; Alzheimer's
- cystitis; high blood levels of urea (indicating kidney malfunction)
- excess platelet count (leading to thrombosis, strokes); high IgE and IgG (antibody) levels resulting from allergies and intolerances
- gallstones; kidney stones
- skin inflammations
- high liver enzymes (indicating poor liver function)
- intraoccular pressure due to excess fluid (sometimes resulting in glaucoma)
- fever
- benign and malignant tumors

Signs of toxicity

Ama can cause blockages in your channels of circulation (e.g., blood clots, constipation), mucus congestion, poor immunity, loss of strength, lack of movement, obstructions to the flow of energy, accumulation of wastes, water retention, bad odors, tense muscles, low digestive fire (*agni*), bloating, diarrhea, itchiness, a thick tongue coating, lack of enthusiasm, and depression. *Ama* physically blocks cosmic intelligence from entering your body–mind and prevents your life force, or *prana*, from helping you to grow. It makes you dull.

How do you become toxic?

Ayurveda states that we can become toxic depending on what we eat and how we digest (*see* Nourishment, pp.39 and 44). When your digestive fire (*agni*) is low, toxins are created. In addition to poor-quality food and contaminated water, we are increasingly exposed to high levels of environmental pollutants and pharmaceutical drugs, which can have a toxic effect on the body.

In keeping with its holistic view of life, Ayurveda extends the idea of poor digestion to our emotional as well as nutritional diet. Increasing levels of stress, extreme emotions, negative images in the media, distressing world events, and the plethora of violence on television, in the cinema, and in computer games all need "digesting" or assimilating, in order to avoid *ama* contaminating the peace and stillness of our consciousness.

But pollution in all its forms is so pervasive that it is virtually impossible not to become overloaded unless you are very disciplined about what you expose yourself to. Once we have started on the toxic path, this can easily become a degenerative cycle, as "like increases like" (see box p.14). Poor digestion leads to further poor digestion. However, the opposite is also true: benevolent cycles of good digestion, healthy tissue creation, and vital essence production (or *ojas*, *see* Rejuvenation, p.111) all coalesce to improve the quality and length of life. This is why it is essential to cleanse regularly.

> ### The top ten toxins
> * Industrial pollutants (dioxins, PCBs, phthalates, heavy metals such as mercury)
> * Pharmaceutical drugs
> * Agricultural pesticides and insecticides
> * Recreational drugs
> * Trans fats and poor-quality oils
> * Intensively farmed meats
> * Refined sugar
> * Nonorganic food
> * Mycotoxins
> * Stress, loneliness, depression

PUKKA PERSPECTIVES

ARE TOXINS REAL?

To anyone practicing natural medicine both the concept and the reality of toxins are very clear. Some corners of mainstream medicine, however, question their existence. Of course, part of this difference is because of the language and perspectives of each tradition; for example, "damp" and "heat" can be thought of as toxins in Ayurveda, just as uric acid or even sugar can become a toxins if too much builds up in the blood (i.e., the terms might be different but the theory is the same). However, some of the contrast between the two schools exists as a result of how traditional and modern medicine differ in their view of health and disease as a whole—and this is the world I want us to examine now.

Whatever perspective you take, a toxin is generally said to be anything that is poisonous and causes damage or death to an organism. Some toxins occur as a result of our everyday biological processes, as mentioned above, while others are generated by external factors, such as when endotoxins are produced in response to bacterial invasion. A good illustration of one that is created in both ways is a substance known as a free radical. Free radicals are potential toxins, as an accumulation can cause inflammation in the body; conventional medicine uses their levels as a measure of overall toxicity. While they occur naturally as the waste products of normal cellular activity, free radicals can also be a response to environmental conditions. So, for example, both aerobic exercise and the inhalation of car exhaust fumes result in their production.

Free radical damage
The body has good mechanisms for neutralizing free radicals, whether they are generated biologically or environmentally. However, when they are present in excessive amounts, free radicals are known to produce negative changes in the body by causing chemical bonds to occur between molecules that are programmed to operate independently. This is known as "cross-linking." These bonds act like a straitjacket, affecting how

cells interact and disrupting the exchange of information between them. A chain reaction ensues. Free radicals damage the formation of the cell membrane and the nucleus, preventing nutrients from moving across the cell membrane. They eat away at the membrane and corrupt its genetic DNA, which alters the evolutionary destiny of the cell. In other words, the cell becomes "sick." This mutation of DNA implicates free radicals in numerous degenerative disorders, from heart disease to Alzheimer's, and from diabetes to cancer. Free radicals literally reduce the ability of cells to adjust to change. And as we are creatures of adaptation, not being able to change can be said to be one of the main causes of disease—a viewpoint that is held by both traditional and mainstream medicine.

Free radical protection

If all this sounds alarming, then it is comforting to note that we are managing the influence of free radicals every day by availing ourselves of antioxidants, accessed in two ways: through the body's own systems of protection and through dietary means. The body's response to free radicals is to generate enzymes known collectively as glutathione peroxidase, which is the major antioxidant produced by cells. Glutathione helps to keep nutritional antioxidants (such as vitamins C and E) in their active forms and it needs sufficient quantities of some trace elements (for example, selenium, copper, and zinc) to be fully functional. The glutathione enzyme is involved in many other cellular roles apart from the neutralization of free radicals, including DNA formation and repair, cellular proliferation, and the maintenance of the immune function. Thus it is an important factor in the aging process: if the level of glutathione in the body drops, the rate of aging increases. Low glutathione levels are most obviously signified by the presence of liver (or "age") spots on the skin, which are also associated with a higher incidence of basal cell carcinoma (the most common type of skin cancer).

The second means of protection is from consuming foods that are themselves rich in antioxidants. Turmeric, green tea, wheat grass juice, grapes, and berries have all been shown to increase glutathione levels, effectively reversing any cellular damage. Antioxidants in vitamins C and E, carotenoids (found in both orange vegetables and dark-green leafy vegetables), and flavonoids (plant pigments) stop us "rusting" so quickly and can help to repair any "corrosion" that has taken place. This is why eating a broad range of brightly colored vegetables is so important: they act to keep your cells healthy, protect your genetic integrit,y and help keep you young.

The detoxification pathways

Detoxification can be defined as a process that removes toxic substances or qualities, whether they are mercury, uric acid, free radicals, or "heat" or "damp," by eliminating them from the system so that a healthful balance, or homeostasis, is found. The liver is a major center of detoxification, as it helps to break down much of what goes into the body, including foods, pharmaceutical drugs, hormones, and industrial pollutants. Other organs, such as the kidneys, bowels, skin, and lungs, as well as the metabolic process of every cell, are equally important. However, a lot of good science has shown how free radicals and other toxins are detoxified through the liver by means of enzymes working in metabolic systems known as the "Phase 1 and Phase 2 detoxification pathways." In essence, these two systems work in tandem to help the body metabolize the levels of potentially harmful substances.

Nevertheless, if excessive amounts are produced, or if your liver function is compromised by other factors in your health, free radicals can overwhelm your body's elimination systems. They literally cause a "traffic jam" in your detoxification pathways. The toxins that the liver cannot metabolize often end up stored in fatty tissue, such as the brain, nerves, and endocrine glands. Hence, natural medicine notes how toxicity, at its most extreme, can be associated with neurological, fertility, metabolic, and energy imbalances.

Why detoxify?

As we have seen, dietary and environmental factors can, at times, compromise the body's defense mechanisms, leading to an overflow of free radicals and other toxins. Traditional systems of health care have used greater purification and cleansing techniques for centuries to take care of the buildup of these toxins. Ayurveda also takes the view that it is equally as important, once the system has been cleansed, to utilize methods of restoring balance and routine.

In summary, whether you look at it from the Ayurvedic point of view of "heat toxins" or "damp toxins" or from the modern position of pollutants and free radicals, toxins are very real. And in the twenty-first century we are now exposed to a greater number than ever before.

SOME COMMON TOXINS

While the body can generate toxins in response to its own metabolic processes, there are a number of substances that we routinely come into contact with that could also fall under the definition of a toxin, due to the detrimental effect they can have on the body.

 ## Alcohol

Although it is popular in many cultures to drink alcohol, it is a renowned toxin, causing liver damage through repeated and excessive exposure. If the liver's detoxification pathways are impaired, a class of compounds called aldehydes, which are formed from alcohol metabolism, can build up to harmful levels and cause damage, since the acids they form are often more toxic than the original substances from which they are derived. The chemical acetaldehyde is one such toxic substance, although it is also one of the impurities found in cheaper wine and spirits. Researchers say that it is probably the metabolism of methanol, the simplest alcohol, to formaldehyde and formic acid that causes the symptoms of the hangover. This is reinforced by the fact that the types of drinks associated with more severe hangovers contain higher levels of methanol: whiskey, cheap red wine, fruit brandy, and other dark spirits. Vodka and other clear drinks contain the least. In the liver, methanol takes ten times longer than ethanol to break down.

 ## Smoking

Smoking in moderation acts as a stimulant that reduces stagnant *kapha* and encourages the appetite. Ayurveda even has some therapeutic treatments involving the smoking of certain medicinal herbs. However, in excess, and especially when the substance is tobacco, smoking aggravates all three *dosha*s and can therefore be considered a toxin. It also leads to a buildup of phlegm in the lungs, as it reduces the efficiency of the mucociliary escalator (the bronchi, throat, and nose), the major barrier for respiratory tract infections—smokers get more coughs and colds. In addition, the hot and dry nature of the smoke can "dry" and harden the mucus, making it more difficult to expectorate.

> Foods for assisting the liver's detoxification pathways
> Those shown in **bold** are particularly beneficial.
> Brassicas (**broccoli**, cauliflower, cabbage, kale, Brussels sprouts, and especially their germinated seed sprouts, which contain high levels of sulforaphane), onion, garlic, **turmeric**, chile, clove, caraway, dill, **rosemary**, orange, tangerine, lemon, foods high in zinc, and vitamins C, B1, and B6. **Milk thistle**, dandelion root, andrographis, and neem also benefit the liver.

Pharmaceutical drugs

Pharmaceutical medications, although designed to be beneficial to our health, can also be toxic (*see* Nourishment, p.42-3). Over two million people a year in the USA are negatively affected by the medication they take, at a cost to hospitals of $76.6 billion due to injury or death. Some consider the modern medical system to be the largest cause of death in developed countries! Just take the example of The Million Women Study in the UK, where Hormone Replacement Therapy (HRT) use in women aged 50 and over is known to have caused an estimated extra 20,000 cases of breast cancer over the decade of its monitoring. Another fact is that one in 1,200 people will die from taking a "painkiller" (e.g., acetaminophen/paracetamol), equivalent to over 1,500 fatalities per year in the UK and approximately 16,500 per year in the USA (making it the fifteenth largest cause of death). A UK study in 2004 put adverse drug reactions (ADRs) at over six percent of all pharmaceutical drug users. Given that the reporting rate is thought to be only twenty-five percent, the actual figure is likely to be much higher. ADRs cause about 10,000 deaths in the UK each year; corticosteroids, anticoagulants, and anticancer medication appear to be most frequently involved. This costs the UK's national health system over $79 million per year in hospitalizations.

> **Foods for helping to clear the lungs**
> Some of the best herbs for the lungs are ginger, pippali, black pepper, licorice, cinnamon, thyme, anise, and marshmallow root. To strengthen the lungs, and to remove dryness, regularly use tonifying foods, such as ghee, almonds (soak overnight and peel the skin), almond milk, pine nuts, tahini (sesame seed butter), and honey. Chywanaprash is an excellent restorative tonic.

Recreational drugs

While some psychotropic drugs can act as short-term catalysts to open new avenues within the body–mind complex, their use can cause imbalances with the *dosha*s. The nature of most drugs is scattering to the life force (*prana*) and depleting to your vital essence, or *ojas*. (For more on this important concept, *see* Rejuvenation, p.111.) This is because they are usually stimulants of some sort, which can push *vata* out to the extremities. Drugs can overly heat the body and are therefore irritating to *pitta*. Many are also diuretics (increase urination) that cause dryness and constipation, and weaken the kidneys. Any drug used excessively tends to damage the groundedness of a person, distorting their mental clarity, and causing dullness and inertia. *See* chart on the next page for herbs which can help counteract the effects of drug use.

Herbs for stabilizing the mind

Those seeking recovery from recreational drug use are advised to consult a qualified practitioner.

Vacha (*Acorus calamus*) Opens the channels of the mind and is invaluable for the treatment of addictions. Only use under guidance from a practitioner.

Turmeric (*Curcuma longa*) Enhances mental circulation.

Gotu kola (*Hydrocotyle asiatica*) Cleanses hallucinogens and the toxins produced by marijuana from the liver and brain.

Ashwagandha (*Withania somnifera*) Rebuilds the nervous system; also reduces anxiety.

Shatavari (*Asparagus racemosus*) Helps restore mental balance and emotional sensitivity.

Valerian (*Valeriana officinalis*) Has natural sedative properties that counteract the long-term effects of stress and stimulants.

Guggul (*Commiphora mukul*) Cleanses and rejuvenates deep tissue; also scrapes away deposits from fat-soluble pesticides from the fatty tissues.

 ## Environmental toxins

Many of the toxins we are exposed to come from the world around us. Many are naturally occurring: mycotoxins (mold), neurotoxins (such as venom), aflatoxins (a type of fungus commonly found on peanuts, spices, and grains, and one of the leading causes of liver cancer). Many more are manmade, and are being produced in increasing amounts: in 1930 we made one million metric tons of chemicals and in 2010 more than 200 million metric tons.

Human-generated toxins are now omnipresent in our environment. The chemical, pharmaceutical, agriculture, and food industries have created a host of toxins that have infiltrated our air, water, and soil. These have unwittingly penetrated our food chain and our homes, and are a part of our ecosystem in the guise of insecticides, pesticides, herbicides, flame-retardants, heavy metals, petrochemicals, pharmaceutical drugs, and radiation. According to the Environmental Protection Agency, more than four billion pounds of toxic compounds were released into the environment in the USA in 2004—double the amount released there in 1994. Despite DDT having been banned in the UK since 1984, traces of this insecticide can still be found in most people today.

And, ironically, we are all dependent on the everyday products from which industrial toxins are derived.

Numerous studies attest to the detrimental effect of the increase in these toxins in our environment on our ecosystem and our health. For example, benzene (used in the chemical industry to make many drugs and plastics) is associated with lymphoma and leukemia, aniline dyes (used for clothing color) are associated with bladder cancer, asbestos with lung cancer, radiation with gene mutation, pesticides with a host of hormonal imbalances leading to different cancers and disruption to wildlife. And few studies have been done on how industrial toxins interact with each other.

The particular troublemakers are endocrine disruptor chemicals (EDCs), so-called because they interfere with the workings of our endocrine system, which influences our hormone balance. EDCs have estrogen-like and antiandrogenic qualities. They mimic natural hormones, inhibiting their action, and altering the normal regulatory function of the endocrine system. This causes imbalances in our reproductive, developmental, behavioral, neurological, and immunological health. And EDCs are everywhere: in plastics, cosmetics, personal care products, cleaning agents, clothing, household furnishings and decorations, food and water, fertilizers, pesticides, and fungicides. They are easily air- and water-borne, leading to widespread contamination in most parts of the globe.

EDCs are fat-soluble and are stored in the body for extended periods of time. Children, the elderly, and those with suppressed immune systems are typically more susceptible to many kinds of pollutants; childhood cancers, such as leukemia, have been associated in particular with fetal exposure to EDCs. Men and women of reproductive age are especially at risk because of the link with impaired fertility and associated problems, such as accelerated puberty, gynecological abnormalities, and premature delivery.

EDCs are members of a larger group of chemicals that were widely used during the industrial boom that followed World War II, now known as persistent organic pollutants (POPs). While POPs had many beneficial effects at the time in pest and disease control, they have since had many unforeseen effects on human health and the environment.

OUR DETOX CULTURE

There is a puritanical streak running through many of the cultural values that we learn when we are young; for example, that the denial of material possessions brings you closer to "God." It's the idea of "no pain, no gain." While it makes some sense, it is not absolutely true. Many religions also deny our flesh, our physicality, and our sexuality. They lock certain emotions away and prohibit certain forms of behavior in favor of what they consider to be "pure." However, we do not need to deny ourselves to be whole. The monastery is not necessarily a place of purity. The healthiest and most spiritual people I have met are not leading "pure" lives but integrated ones. They are not denying life but accepting it. They are honoring who they are, rather than who they have been told they should be.

Our society has an unhealthy view of the body, perceiving it as toxic and dirty. We only have to consider our imbalanced relationship with dieting or the huge sales in laxatives to see that this is the case. Despite what many belief systems claim, we are not inherently "toxic." We are exposed to a host of toxic environmental pollutants, our food is denatured and our digestive and nervous systems extremely challenged. But that does not mean we have to detox constantly. Even if your lifestyle is pretty good, you may be building up toxins because your system is not strong enough to metabolize them. In that case you may just need some tonics to boost your strength in order to cleanse efficiently (*see* Rejuvenation, p.122). We sometimes need to clean and we sometimes need to build, often at the same time, but rarely in isolation or continuously. It is all about finding a balance.

One of the things I love about Ayurveda is that it is not concerned with what is good or bad. Following its practices does not involve denying yourself a treat or a drink (or whatever your preference might be); it's about learning about who you are, what you need, and being true to yourself. And, in my experience, this changes from moment to moment. This is your goal: to learn what is right for you, at any stage in time—no "shoulds," just choices that serve you.

THE AYURVEDIC THEORY OF ILLNESS

Before we can fully understand why cleansing is so beneficial to our health, we should consider the nature of illness and the course it takes in the body. Ayurveda approaches this in a typically holistic and metaphorical manner. It says that along with external factors, such as genetic diseases, traumatic accidents, and *karmic* reasons (the effect on us from previous actions), illness has four primary causes: crimes against wisdom; restraining your natural urges; unwholesome attachment of your senses to their objects; and seasonal influences.

The phrase "crimes against wisdom" means to deny our intuition and ignore our past experiences; for example, acting inappropriately for what you really need or not learning from our mistakes. This could include eating what we know is not good for us, or behaving in a way that leads to conflict. It's the sort of thing that usually gets us into trouble.

When I consider the meaning of "restraining your natural urges,", it conjures up memories of when I was younger and having to hold back the giggles when I definitely should not have been laughing. Of course, this doesn't hurt, but regularly holding back our natural functions leads to repression of the body's energy flow. Ayurveda points out that thirst, hunger, sneezing, yawning, crying, urinating, defecating, farting, burping, orgasm, sleeping, waking, and panting due to overexertion should never be restrained. It teaches that withholding any of these functions leads to various stagnations and blockages, resulting in headaches, pain, bloating or, more seriously, dizziness, fainting, and even death. But this is not a license to indulge and it's important to maintain a balance.

When we strongly like or dislike something, we display an "unwholesome attachment of the senses to their objects." The overuse or inappropriate application of the senses, such as desiring something too much, too little, or when inappropriate for your constitution, can unbalance your *dosha*, leading to illness. Ayurvedic teachings emphasize that moderation in all things is essential for perfect health.

The phrase "seasonal influences" describes common and predictable patterns that disturb our health and make us unwell: spring flu, summer allergies, fall aches, and winter colds. In my practice I always see more eczema in the spring, hives in the summer, insomnia in the fall, and depression in the winter. When you understand why they occur, you can protect yourself against these seasonal tendencies (*see* Ecology, p.197).

THE PATHWAY OF DISEASE

Impaired digestion/low *agni*

Disease manifests with
unique characteristics

Imbalance is
disturbed

Disease arises

Imbalance spreads,
toxins spill over

Aggravated *doshas* move
to other sites

The learned Ayurvedic doctors of the past worked out a six-stage pathway that describes the progression of many acute and chronic illnesses, showing how a few minor symptoms can turn into a full-blown disease.

When digestion is faulty and digestive fire (*agni*) is low, an imbalance builds up in a place associated with the particular *dosha*: *vata* imbalances start to collect in the large intestine; *pitta* accumulates in the small intestine; *kapha* gathers in the stomach. Illnesses occurring at this stage, such as constipation, stomach acidity, or sluggish digestion, are relatively easy to remove, but if it is not addressed quickly, the situation can deteriorate.

The second stage of disease progression is when the imbalance becomes disturbed. If the causes continue, then the aggravated *dosha*—the imbalance of *vata, pitta,* or *kapha*—will start to irritate the organs; a *dosha* can be a friend or foe, depending on its levels, so here the increased *dosha* in a sense becomes a toxin. At this stage of the pathway, the aggravation is still relatively easy to remove via the digestive tract.

Next, if left untreated, the imbalance spreads. Having reached maximum capacity in their respective sites, the accumulated and aggravated toxins now cross their threshold and spill over into other parts of the body. They move out of the digestive tract and spread to other associated locations via the blood and lymph. With *vata* they spread to the skin causing dryness, to the joints causing cracking and pain, to the air passages causing a dry cough, and to the intestines causing further pain and obstructed peristaltic motions. With *pitta* they move to the skin causing inflammatory skin problems, to the eyes causing redness, to the stomach causing nausea, and to the bowels causing burning diarrhea. With *kapha* they spread to the lungs causing a wet cough, breathing difficulties, and vomiting, to the joints causing swelling, and to the bowel causing mucus in the stool. However, even at this late stage the toxins are still relatively easy to clear from the system.

During the fourth stage the illness becomes more apparent. The aggravated *dosha*s settle in a fixed location, either in an area of weakness or in one of the areas of the body that the particular *dosha* is associated with: *vata* in the ears, joints, bones, skin, or colon; *pitta* in the liver, eyes, skin, intestinal lining, or glands; *kapha* in the lungs, stomach, joints, mucous membranes, and fluid parts of the body. This is when the signs of disease develop. The *dosha*s are now difficult to clear and require deep cleansing techniques.

During the fifth stage a real disease arises, manifesting as a pathology with a specific set of characteristics and a defined name, such as diabetes or asthma. When the *dosha* has penetrated this deeply and mutated so far from its normal healthy balance, finding a cure is often difficult.

And then we arrive at the sixth and final stage of disease, where it expresses its own unique characteristics. Once a disease is fixed in a particular place it takes on a life of its own; its dominant features are reflected by the primary causative *dosha* and often involve the other *dosha*s, too. For example, eczema is dry, fissured, and itchy when caused by *vata*; red, inflamed, bleeding, and hot when caused by *pitta*; and wet, suppurating, itchy, and edematous when caused by *kapha*. The disease is now chronic; sometimes it becomes incurable.

But the remedy, at least in the early stages, is usually near at hand: clear the "toxins" from your system and come back within the safety of your threshold. The qualities of cold, heat, dry, and damp can become toxic if they build up (*see* p.74), and the best way to rectify this is to eliminate them via the bowels, bladder, stomach, lungs, skin, and, for women, via the uterus with the monthly period. The classic herbal laxatives (encouraging bowel motions), diuretics (encouraging urination), emetics (encouraging vomiting), expectorants (encouraging clearing of mucus), diaphoretics (encouraging sweating), and emmenagogues (encouraging menstruation) help to do this. In the past, some of these practices were called "heroic," as they were used at high doses to cause extreme cleansing, but these days herbalism has developed a much more gentle approach.

CLEANSING THE AYURVEDIC WAY

We cleanse by helping our body–mind to metabolize wastes so that our whole system is kept in balance. We can start to feel symptoms of toxicity when our system is overloaded and our threshold is reached. The idea of a threshold is an important one in Ayurveda. Imagine that your constitutional strength is contained within a vase. When we are born that vase is half full, but as we age and add various elements of diet, life, and our environment into that vase, it can fill up. As it fills up we start to experience some minor symptoms, but when it completely fills up and overflows then real illness can start. If we can keep the levels below the top of the vase, as if it has a faucet in the bottom to let wastes out, then we can stay in balance. This is our daily challenge.

An occasional detoxification can put a bounce in your step and a sparkle in your eyes. It should leave you clearheaded and relaxed, so you sleep soundly and feel refreshed upon waking. The best times of year to detoxify are at the junctions of the seasons in the early spring and early fall, in order to cleanse the accumulated mucus from winter and the dry heat from the summer. It will invigorate you so that you are ready to enjoy the wonders of each season with renewed health and enthusiasm.

While detoxification cleanses your system, it is important also to rebalance (*see* next page), nourish, and rejuvenate (*see* Rejuvenation, p.100) properly afterward: there is no point in stripping your system and leaving it vulnerable. Remember that if you are very ill, pregnant, or elderly, you should never do a cleansing without the guidance of a practitioner, if at all. For details of cleansing herbs, *see* p.92.

Cleansing your bowels

Although a good diet naturally maintains digestive health, it is wise to undertake a regular bowel cleanse in order to completely detoxify your system. The Ayurvedic formula triphala is a mix of three fruits that are famed for their ability to mildly detoxify the bowel. It is also important to keep the strength of your digestive fire (*agni*) strong, so remember to include herbs and spices such as ginger, black pepper, cumin, coriander, and fennel in your diet.

Cleansing your liver

As the major organ of detoxification, the liver qualifies for special attention. Bitter foods, such as artichoke leaf, dandelion root, chicory root, and turmeric, can help the liver do its job more effectively, as can the medicinal "pukka" herbs andrographis and gotu kola (*see also* p.78). Neem leaf is a famous Ayurvedic herb that can help regulate the flow of bile, protect the liver and encourage regeneration of liver cells. Aloe vera juice is one of the best tonics for cooling and nourishing liver function.

Cleansing your lungs

 Remedies for lung problems focus on clearing phlegm, reducing heat, and nourishing the lungs, removing the sticky, hot, dry, and depleting effects of smoking or infections. Trikatu, a combination of ginger, black pepper, and long pepper, is very effective for clearing phlegm and helping to strengthen the lungs. In addition to using herbs and tonifying foods (*see* box, p.79), a powerful way to cleanse your lungs is to practice a special breathing exercise called "the brain-cleansing breath"—*see* the next page for specific instructions. This also increases metabolism and oxygen supply to the brain, awakening the mind and revitalizing your whole system.

Hot water
One of the simplest cleansing tools is always close to hand and costs very little. Hot water is a wonderful medicine that strengthens digestion and is a great cleanser. Think of washing up: if you have a greasy plate and you use cold water, the fat will simply congeal. However, if you use warm water, the grease will melt away. Drink this freely throughout the day.

Cleansing your skin

The skin is a good indicator of how well your body is eliminating wastes. Skin blemishes, such as acne or boils, can be a sign that the bowels, liver, and kidneys are not removing wastes properly, forcing the body to remove them via the skin. They could also indicate that your elimination system is overloaded with too many toxins. Herbs such as neem, guduchi, turmeric, chamomile, nettles, and burdock root and seed are known to alter the chemistry of your tissues, bringing them back to optimum function through helping the lymph, liver, kidneys, and intercellular fluid rebalance. If you take the herbs with aloe vera it will have a stronger effect, as aloe vera is a "carrier" to the skin.

Another useful cleansing treatment for the skin is self-massage. Rub yourself from head to foot with scant ½ cup of warm sesame oil. Leave on for ten minutes, then wash off in a hot bath or shower. This will dilate the pores, allowing toxins to be cleared through the skin and, by helping congested lymph to return to the heart, enables any residual toxins to be excreted via the liver and kidneys. *See* Strength and Stillness, p.170 for more details on massage.

The brain-cleansing breath (*kapalabhati*)

This breathing technique involves strongly expelling the air from your lungs and allowing the natural relaxation following this contraction to draw fresh air back in, like a sponge naturally regaining its shape after being squeezed. While it is safe for almost everyone, it's always best to have the guidance of a yoga teacher, and should not be done by anyone who suffers from high blood pressure, vertigo, or hernias.

Sit comfortably in a cross-legged position. Allow the body to ground, the spine to be straight, mouth to close, eyes to lightly shut, and the breath to settle. Become aware of your breath flowing in and out. When you are ready, start to expel the air in your lungs forcefully through your nostrils, keeping your mouth closed. Concentrate on contracting your abdominal muscles and drawing your stomach in. This moves your diaphragm upward and inward, pushing the stale air out from your lungs. When all of the breath is out, allow your stomach to relax. This will draw your diaphragm down and bring in fresh air.

Breathe in and out quite quickly, having a breath each second. Repeat 25 to 50 times and then draw a deep breath in and hold for a few moments before breathing out.

Breathe normally for a few breaths and, when you feel ready, repeat the whole practice three to five times. Your lungs will now be cleansed, your blood rid of higher levels of carbon dioxide and replenished with fresh oxygen and life force (*prana*).

DAILY CONSTITUTIONAL BALANCING

While we need to have regular times of "cleansing," we can reduce the need for more extreme detoxification by taking care of ourselves every day. This involves all the fundamentals of healthy Ayurvedic living: tending to your digestive fire (*agni*); caring for your constitutional *dosha*; adjusting your lifestyle to the weather and the season; and, most importantly, living according to how you feel. For specific diets to aid the balancing of the *dosha*s, *see* Nourishment, p.64.

Balancing your digestive fire (*agni*)

There is a traditional Ayurvedic saying that states, "All diseases are caused by an under-functioning digestive system." A balanced digestive fire is key to optimum digestion, and the best advice for achieving this is to follow your body. Listen to what your digestive system is telling you. Notice how you feel before you eat: are you really hungry? How do you feel once you have eaten: heavy or energized? Be aware of how you digest certain foods. If you can allow your inner intelligence to guide you, then you will be more likely to find out what is truly healthy and right for you. Move slowly with this awareness and learn at a pace that suits you.

Try to eat only when hungry, gently stoking the digestive fire with digestible meals. Avoid smothering your *agni* with foods that are excessively cold, damp, or heavy, or aggravating

How to balance your digestive fire (*agni*)

A few Ayurvedic dietary guidelines can give you a head start in learning what is good for your digestion.

* Leave 4 to 6 hours between meals. The sign that the previous meal is digested is when you feel light and your breath is fresh.
* Don't snack between meals, provided that your blood sugar is stable, as this slows your digestion. Try drinking some herbal tea or warm water when you feel hungry.
* Minimize foods with cold, wet, and heavy qualities, as they weaken digestion.
* Drink hot water, ginger tea, or spicy teas to stimulate digestion.
* Eat an "aperitif" of bitter-tasting foods to increase the secretion of hydrochloric acid in the stomach (useful for *kapha* types).
* Use a small dose (0.5–1g) of stimulating, digestive herbs before a meal. Some of the best are ginger, black pepper, pippali (long pepper), cumin, clove, cinnamon, and fennel.
* Start a meal with spicy, sour, and salty flavors, as these increase *agni*.
* Do not overeat or undereat, as both disrupt your digestive energy.

it with excessively spicy, oily, or fried foods. There are also many preconceptions about food that you will have to face and unlearn. For example, yogurt is generally considered to be a healthy food, but its "dampness" can cause mucus and congestion—more so when eaten in a cold, damp winter straight from the refrigerator. Fruit is also seen as beneficial, but it is important to leave some time before eating other foods, as it can cause fermentation (*see* Nourishment, p.55). Choose what is in season and what grows in your own climate—it can reduce the impact of seasonal change. Following nature's wisdom can be a great help on the path to balance. *See* the box above for some further tips.

Balancing light *vata*

As we have seen, *vata* is aggravated by astringent, bitter, and pungent flavors (as they all increase dryness), at the end of a meal, in the early morning and evening, by fear and insecurity, in early fall and spring, at the latter stage of life, by excessive movement, by a dry and cold climate, by going to bed after 11pm. If out of balance, there is a natural tendency for *vata* types to be attracted to these destabilizing influences. As *vata* is light, cold, dry, it is best balanced by using the opposite qualities: groundedness, warmth, moisture.

Reduce these experiences:
* bitter, astringent or pungent foods (cold salads, black tea, very hot spices)
* rushing, traveling
* cold, dryness
* fear, anxiety

Include more of these experiences:
* warm oil massage: use sesame oil, mahanarayan oil, *vata* oil
* oily, soupy, and heavy foods
* regularity: a daily routine is essential
* warmth: hot water, warm clothes, and environment, warming herbal teas and spices
* stillness: learn relaxation techniques and calm yoga practices
* confidence and security: enhance self-esteem and positive thinking

Vata treatment concentrates on regulating the lower abdomen and clearing dryness and tension from the bowels to ensure nervous toxins move out of the body. Use digestive carminatives to reduce gas and demulcent laxatives and enemas to soften stools. Licorice, triphala, flaxseeds, and ginger are all helpful for either strengthening digestion or warming it up. Then tone the nervous system using nourishing "pukka" herbs, such as ashwagandha, shatavari, and chywanaprash.

Balancing hot *pitta*

Pitta is aggravated by pungent, salty, and sour flavors (as they increase heat), in the middle of a meal, at midday, by anger and irritation, repressed emotions, in summer, from adolescence to middle age, from excessive ambition, a hot and damp climate. If out of balance, *pitta* types will seek more of the destabilizing elements familiar to them. As *pitta* is hot, oily, and intense, it is best balanced by their opposites: coolness, calmness, loving, compassion, and moderation.

Reduce these experiences:
* pungent, salty, sour foods (chile, spices, salt, fermented foods)
* aggression, competition
* hot environments

Include more of these experiences:

* ❧ sweet, bitter, and astringent foods: grains, fruits, asparagus, lettuce
* ❧ cooling drinks: aloe vera juice, rosewater, cold peppermint tea, drinking yogurt flavored with coriander, wheatgrass juice
* ❧ calming massage with light oils: almond, coconut, grapeseed, *pitta* oil
* ❧ compassionate meditation and uncompetitive yoga

Pitta is generally alleviated by clearing heat from the digestive system, liver, and the blood. Use mild laxatives and blood-cleansing herbs such as amla, neem leaf, or triphala, followed by nourishing but cooling tonics, such as aloe vera, shatavari, licorice and wheatgrass juice. The microalgae superfoods spirulina and chlorella are also good for keeping *pitta* within its heat threshold.

Balancing heavy *kapha*

Kapha is aggravated by sweet, sour, and salty flavors (as they increase moisture), at the beginning of a meal, in the morning (7–11am) and evening (7–11pm), by greed and possessiveness, in winter, by a cold, heavy and damp diet, in childhood, by a damp and cold climate, by sleeping in the day, by lack of movement and laziness. Again, because "like increases like," there is a natural tendency for *kapha* types to be attracted to the qualities that tip them out of balance. As *kapha* is slow, damp, and heavy, it is best balanced with the opposite: movement and activity, dryness, lightness.

Reduce these experiences:

* ❧ sweet, sour, salty foods (sugar, yogurt, salt)
* ❧ cold, refrigerated, damp, wet food (ice, dairy, out-of-season fruits)
* ❧ laziness

Include more of these experiences:

* ❧ bitter, astringent, and pungent foods (asparagus, black tea, spices)
* ❧ exercise, dynamic behavior: practice Ashtanga yoga, metabolic exercise
* ❧ giving, sharing, letting go
* ❧ heat, saunas, deep massage with drying powders, mustard oil, *kapha* oil
* ❧ drinks of hot water and spicy teas.

Kapha is best treated by focusing on clearing mucus from the stomach and lungs. Use expectorants, such as pippali, ginger, black pepper, or trikatu. Then use warming herbs and tonics such as ashwagandha, cinnamon, and chywanaprash.

THE BEST CLEANSING HERBS

Traditional health systems around the world all use a plethora of detoxifying herbs, and Ayurveda has its own favorites. However, each plant needs to be used appropriately for each person, at the right time, and in the correct amount. Effectively, this means that there is a huge range of cleansing herbs to choose from and you would be best advised to seek the help of a qualified practitioner in order to gain maximum benefit. The following are some of the principle herbs used for detoxification in Ayurveda (*see* The Pukka Pantry for full details of each).

Digestive cleansers

Ginger (*Zingiber officinale*) Ginger is also known as *vishwa-bheshaja* in Sanskrit, meaning "the universal medicine," as it benefits everybody and all health imbalances, especially "cold" and nervous *vata* disorders. Ginger's warming and drying properties can be your best friend in times of need. Pungent in taste, ginger stimulates the secretion of digestive enzymes, aiding the elimination of toxins. Use fresh ginger in your cooking or as a tea.

Triphala Blended from three nourishing fruits (haritaki, bibhitaki, and amla), the triphala formula is high in antioxidants and performs the functions of healing perfectly. It also has potent cleansing effects, particularly for the digestive tract,

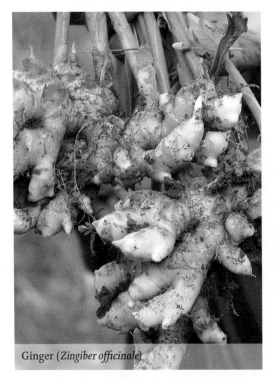

Ginger (*Zingiber officinale*)

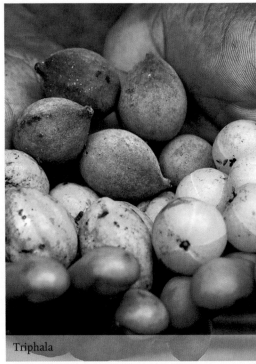

Triphala

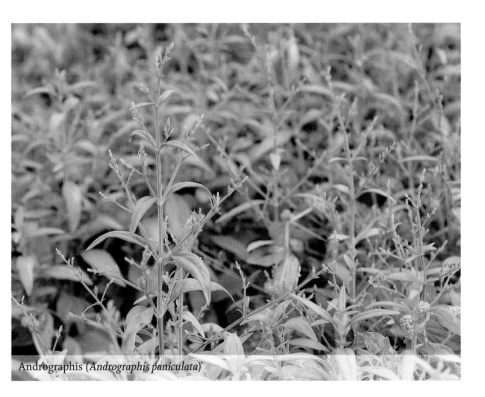
Andrographis (*Andrographis paniculata*)

where it is used for sluggish bowels, constipation, bloating, flatulence, abdominal pain, and indigestion. It can help to heal ulcers, inflammation, hemorrhoids, and general dysbiosis in the gastrointestinal tract. If you are regularly constipated, mix with some psyllium husk to bring moisture into your bowels. Triphala can be used long-term, as its healing effects improve with time.

Liver cleansers
Andrographis (*Andrographis paniculata*) Also known as *mahatikta*, or "the king of bitters" due to its extremely bitter taste, andrographis has an exceptional liver-protecting ability. Use it when your liver is under stress: after drinking alcohol or taking pharmaceutical drugs, or after overexposure to environmental pollutants or viruses.

Lung cleansers
Trikatu Made from equal parts of dry ginger, black pepper, and pippali (long pepper), this Ayurvedic formula rejuvenates the lungs and helps to clear mucus. Use for asthma, bronchitis, pneumonia, coughs, and colds, or whenever there is breathing difficulty or wheezing.

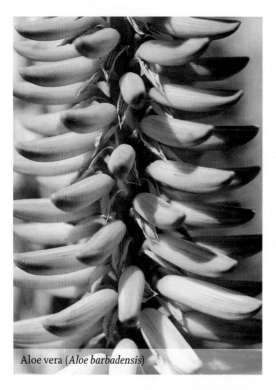

Aloe vera (*Aloe barbadensis*)

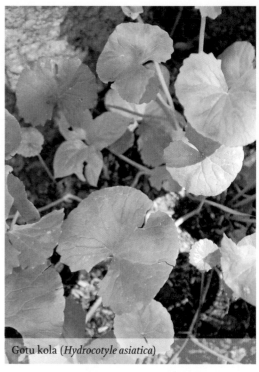

Gotu kola (*Hydrocotyle asiatica*)

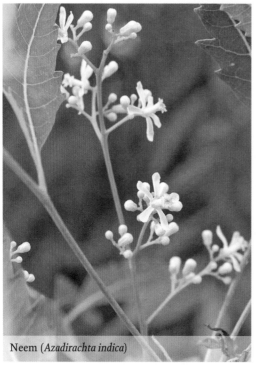

Neem (*Azadirachta indica*)

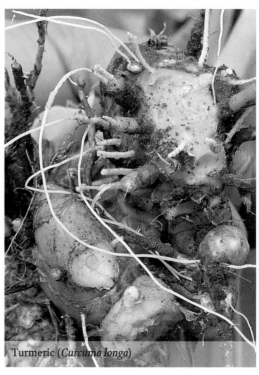

Turmeric (*Curcuma longa*)

Discovering the True You with Ayurveda

Skin and blood cleansers

Aloe vera juice (*Aloe barbadensis*) Aloe vera is a wonderful intestinal healer and skin tonic that nourishes, soothes, and heals when used either internally or externally. It also makes medication taste a little more pleasant and is a good "messenger" for transporting tonic herbs to the deeper tissues, making the individual ingredients more effective than when used alone. For example, shatavari and aloe vera juice synergize when combined.

Gotu kola (*Hydrocotyle asiatica*) Gotu kola has renowned blood-cleansing properties in Ayurveda and is used extensively for inflammatory skin diseases. Take whenever there is redness, swelling, and itching.

Neem (*Azadirachta indica*) In addition to its function as a liver cleanser, neem is one of Ayurveda's primary plants for clearing heat, reducing inflammation, and purifying the blood. As such, it is used for the treatment of skin conditions such as eczema, psoriasis, and acne.

Joint cleansers

Boswellia (*Boswellia serrata*) Also known as Indian frankincense, boswellia is a powerful bitter and pungent-tasting resin used to reduce pain, wounds and inflammation. It has a special "scraping" property that removes toxic adhesions and deposits from joints and the channels, and is useful for relieving rheumatoid arthritis and osteoarthritis.

Turmeric (*Curcuma longa*) Ayurveda considers that the ability of turmeric to clear the blood of toxins can help to purify the skin, prevent pain, stop menstrual pain, reduce rheumatoid arthritis and, specifically, stop shoulder pain. Use liberally in your cooking.

Mind cleansers

Brahmi (*Bacopa monnieri*) Brahmi is a wonderful cooling herb for the nervous system and mind, helping to promote clear thinking. Take whenever there are any signs of mental or emotional imbalance resulting in nervous anxiety or debility.

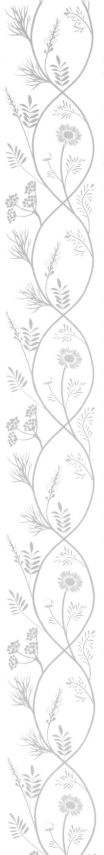

PUKKA PRACTICE

SEASONAL DETOXIFICATION AND FASTING

Because we all accumulate toxins, a gentle seasonal detoxification will be beneficial, whatever your constitution. Depending on your lifestyle, you can choose a fairly simple weekend detox or a more dedicated seven-day regime.

Although not always an immediately popular choice, fasting is a very effective way to detoxify. It helps the digestive system to rest and to let go of attachments to food, and the mind to be at ease and become peaceful.

Remember that Ayurveda is not just about taking appropriate remedies—it is a whole lifestyle.

So, when following any cleansing regime:
❀ eat a simple, organic diet (avoid processed foods, sugar, yeast, nonorganic dairy, and hydrogenated oils)
❀ take plenty of rest
❀ reduce strenuous exercise; practice a gentle form of yoga instead
❀ have a massage or go to a steam room to sweat toxins out; do a daily self-massage
❀ avoid the news and TV to keep media toxins to a minimum

Your seasonal detoxification diet

Try this for a week around the time of the spring equinox (March 21st) and/or fall equinox (September 21st). Base your diet on the principles listed below and emphasize pungent, bitter, astringent flavors (*see* Nourishment, pp.51–3).

Grains No bread or pastries. Less wheat and oats. Take kicharee (*see* next page), barley, quinoa, millet, rye, basmati rice.
Beans Mung beans are best.
Vegetables Steamed sprouts and vegetables (some raw is good for *pitta*). Lots of greens: broccoli, spinach, kale. No mushrooms, root, or excessively sweet vegetables.
Fruits No sweet fruit, only sour, such as cranberry, lemon, lime, grapefruit.
Nuts and seeds No nuts; some pumpkin seeds.
Meat and fish No shellfish, fish, red meat, pork, or associated meat fats.
Dairy None, including eggs; some goat milk can be taken, as it is slightly astringent and less *kapha*-forming; ghee is fine in small quantities.
Oils None, although small amounts of mustard or flaxseed oil (which are drying) are fine.
Herbs and spices Take triphala at night with some warm water. Also take some cleansing herbs during the day.
Sweeteners None (sugar is *ama*-forming). Honey is fine (max. 2 teaspoons per day).
Superfoods Microalgae, especially chlorella.
Drinks No coffee or black tea; take ginger, cinnamon, cardamom, and fennel teas, or dandelion root coffee.

Fasting

A fast leaves you feeling lighter, refreshed, and energized, with clear skin and bright eyes. There are several types, whereby all but the named foodstuff is omitted from the diet: water, fruit juice, rice, soup, kicharee. When you fast, it is important to put some time and thought into it and do it in a way that is appropriate for your constitutional blueprint. As always, you should apply the general wisdom of Ayurveda to your unique and specific needs.

Most importantly, during a fast remember to:
* drink lots of warm water
* drink spicy teas to help "burn" toxins: cinnamon, ginger, clove
* sleep at regular times and for a regular length
* avoid all overstimulation: news, radio, newspapers; reduce social activities
* take a mild laxative, such as triphala or a little castor oil (1 teaspoon), during the fast to help clear toxins from the system
* break your fast slowly: one day of fasting requires one day of reintroducing simple foods

The *vata* fast

Vata types naturally have difficulty in holding on to energy, and so they need to take extra care when undertaking a fast. They already have too little body weight and have a tendency to be ungrounded, so should avoid limiting their much-needed nutrition for too long as this will cause further imbalance. If you are a *vata* type, you should only fast for a short time—between one and three days—and your fast should always contain some simple nourishment, such as rice, mung-bean soup, or kicharee (*see* the next page for recipes). This type of "monofast" calms the mind and kindles the digestive fire (*agni*) without weakening the body.

The *pitta* fast

Pitta types are good at managing energy, have balanced weight but have a tendency to build up inflammatory heat toxins. They can benefit from a fast of one to three days and can manage on appropriate fruit or vegetable juices. A mung-bean soup fast can also be good for *pitta* types. Take account of how busy you are—you must rest, no matter how difficult you find it, to avoid becoming depleted.

The *kapha* fast

Kapha types store energy and tend to be overweight and too static. They can tolerate longer fasts and gain most benefit from them. If you are a *kapha* type, your fast can be based either on a light mung-bean soup or even just hot water and spicy teas. This will stimulate your metabolism to throw off old deposits, and bring lightness and clarity into your whole system.

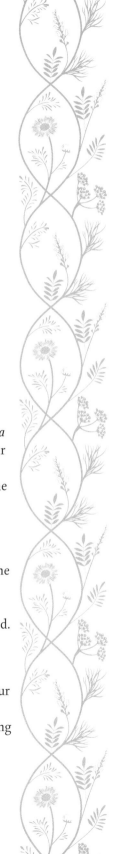

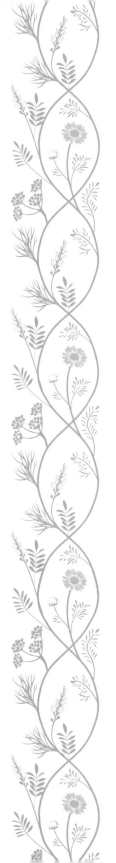

Kicharee

This dish, also known as "food of the gods," is a little like curried risotto, but easier to make. It is an all around healing and digestion-kindling meal.

(makes 2–3 portions)
½ cup split mung beans (or other lentil)
½ cup basmati rice (or other grain, such as quinoa or brown rice)
Ghee or oil
1-inch piece fresh ginger, minced
1 teaspoon cumin seeds
1 teaspoon mustard seeds
3–4 cups water
$^1/_2$ teaspoon Seagreens seaweed mix
$^1/_4$ teaspoon each of turmeric, ginger powder, coriander powder
Pinch of asafetida powder
A few seasonal vegetables (chopped if necessary)
1 teaspoon hemp-seed oil (or ghee)
Sea salt, to taste
Handful of fresh cilantro
Roasted seeds, e.g., sesame
Fresh chutney (optional)

Wash the mung beans and rice. Heat the ghee or oil in a heavy-bottom pan and fry the fresh ginger, cumin, and mustard seeds. Add the mung beans and rice along with the water (a ratio of 1:3 or 1:4), bring to a boil then gently simmer for about 20 minutes. Next, add the seaweed mix, followed by the turmeric, ginger, cilantro, and asafetida. Finally add the seasonal vegetables: spinach, peas, carrots, or shiitake mushrooms work well.

Turn the heat down to low, cover the pan and cook for 10 to 20 minutes. Do not stir until the liquid is nearly absorbed or it will go mushy.

After cooking, add a teaspoon of hemp-seed oil or ghee, and salt to taste. Sprinkle with fresh cilantro and roasted seeds, and serve. Eat with some fresh chutney, if desired.

Mung-bean soup

This simple soup is nourishing, delicious, and easy to make.

(makes 4 portions)
2 cups mung beans
2½ cups water
2-inch piece washed seaweed (kombu) or a sprinkle of Seagreens seaweed mix
1 teaspoon ground cumin
½ teaspoon turmeric
3 tablespoons ghee or virgin coconut oil for frying
1 teaspoon each cumin seed, coriander seed, fennel seed, and mustard seed
1-inch piece ginger (freshly chopped)
¼ teaspoon asafetida powder
1 pinch salt
Handful of fresh cilantro

Soak the mung beans for 4 to 12 hours. Drain, then add fresh water and simmer for 40 minutes with some washed seaweed, ground cumin, and turmeric. Top off with more water if the mixture becomes too dry. In a separate pan heat the ghee or oil and fry the cumin, coriander, fennel and high heat until brown. Add the ginger and asafoetida and cook for a few seconds until you can smell the spicy aroma. Pour this spiced oil into the soup and simmer for another 10 minutes. Add a pinch of salt and sprinkle with fresh cilantro to serve.

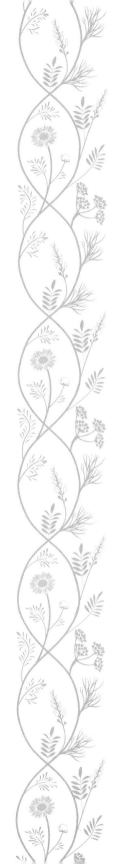

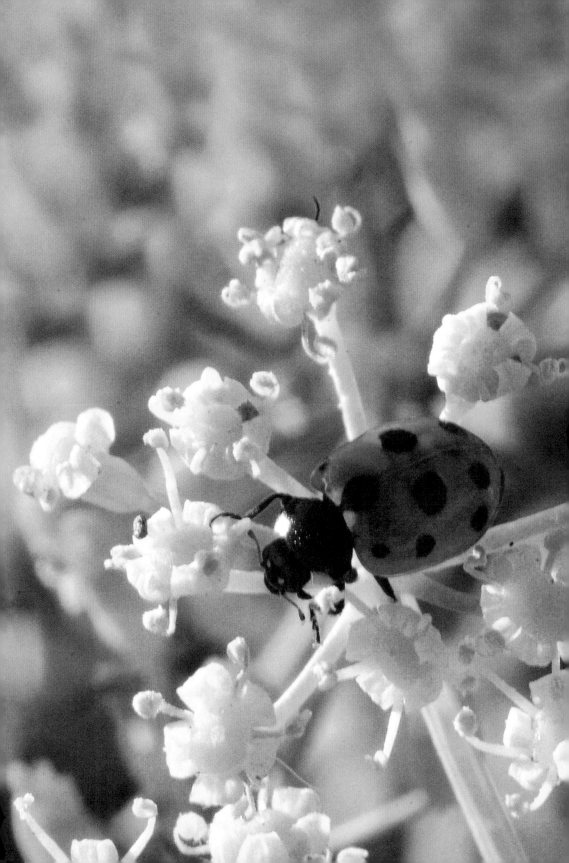

4 REJUVENATION

> **"***Rejuvenation brings you a long life, a sharp memory, intelligence, freedom from disease, youthfulness, beauty, a sweet voice, respect and brilliance.***"**
> **CHARAKA SAMHITA**

We all want to feel great and, quite simply, life is more difficult when we don't feel at our best. How we can keep moving toward this goal is constantly to renew and replenish our health. This process is called rejuvenation, known as *rasayana* in Ayurveda, or "the path of juice." Following rejuvenative practices hastens recovery from disease, improves your mind and intellect, promotes longevity, and delays the symptoms of old age—"to rejuvenate" literally means "to make young again." Some gerontologists think that we should, and easily could, live to be over a hundred. Wouldn't that be amazing? But successful rejuvenation requires an understanding of how your life works as one whole and how you can sustain that through the practices of Ayurveda. Only then can your immunity, heart, digestion, hormones, nervous system, and emotions dance together in one smooth waltz.

THE NEW YOU

Just imagine feeling full of energy, bursting with vitality, having bright eyes, clear skin, excellent digestion, a quick healing response, healthy desires, and being full of optimism. Now imagine the opposite—it's a bit bleak. Up to the age of twenty we have a growing "*kapha*" phase that is anabolic and full of energy and abundance; from twenty to about 60 we enter a more catabolic "*pitta*" phase, where we find repair and regeneration progressively more difficult; and from 60 onward, if we haven't looked after ourselves, we creak all the way until the end of the road.

Rejuvenation—the Ayurvedic context

Good immunity and rejuvenation comes from:
- balancing your constitutional *dosha*
- balancing your digestion
- keeping the channels of circulation open
- having a strong heart and balanced emotions
- nourishing the tissues and organs
- avoiding the causes of poor immunity
- reducing levels of toxicity
- avoiding negative habits and behavioral patterns that can reduce your inherent vitality

Being able to rejuvenate means having access to:
- pure air
- pure water
- pure food
- emotional stability: love, peace of mind, balanced relationships
- a regular lifestyle
- protection: daily activities should be healing, focusing on eating foods to keep your immune system intact and avoiding immune-depressing chemicals
- detoxification: daily, seasonal, and whenever required; deep purification if there is strength, gentle purification in more depleted states; daily regulation of the elimination of toxins
- tonification: daily and seasonal integration of tonifying herbs, foods, yoga practices
- rejuvenating herbs and foods: sweet in taste, juicy in essence, and rejuvenating in effect

One measure of our health is how effectively the immune system works. We know that the majority of health imbalances affect our immunity in one way or another, and that immunity is also compromised by living a life where we give out more than we put back. If we want to turn back the clock—in other words, rejuvenate—we need to reverse this process of decline with regular "top-ups" that help us to replenish. This can be a vacation, a yoga class, a massage, or nourishing time with friends and family. But the real secret to rejuvenation is in your daily routine.

Ayurveda lays much emphasis on prevention in order to avoid the degenerative cascade that can occur when the threshold of our health is breached. The foundation of prevention is an orderly routine that balances personal hygiene, nourishment, exercise, relaxation, creativity, wealth, and love. You can therefore optimize your rejuvenation on a daily basis by regulating your lifestyle, diet, herbal supplements, and emotional habits. Rejuvenating your immunity will truly help to create a new you: the *true* you.

WHAT IS IMMUNITY?

Immunity is the body's defense against infections. It is also part of healthy homeostasis, the dynamic process that the body engages with to stay in balance; it maintains the relationship between our mental, physical, and spiritual selves, our life, and the world in which we live and interact. Immunity should therefore be seen as a holistic system involving our inner and outer worlds. In addition, the immune system is connected to our psychological, neurological, and endocrine systems; in other words, our emotional, nervous, and hormonal responses all communicate with each other to optimize our health. And facilitating healthy communication between these different areas of our life is the key to healthy immunity. As a reflection of this multidimensional activity, our immune system requires nourishment from diverse sources.

You don't need to be a doctor to understand that our immune systems are facing a unique historical challenge as we encounter increased environmental, social, pharmaceutical, dietary, and spiritual stress. And as the global population increases and the industrial world expands, many ecosystems are becoming destabilized, putting the earth's natural "immunity" under stress. We now know that the causes of environmental change and demands of our modern lifestyles can have a negative impact on our own immune systems and overall health, too. A sick world makes for sick people. And vice versa. Our personal challenge is a reflection of the larger environmental one: how can we weave our way through this maze to create both a healthy inner and outer world?

HOW THE IMMUNE SYSTEM WORKS

In order to protect us from foreign invaders (antigens), such as bacteria and viruses, our immune system must be able to differentiate "self" from "nonself." To fulfil, this objective the immune system galvanizes numerous cells, organs, and chemicals to work cooperatively in protecting us against disease. There are two main divisions in your immune system: natural immunity and acquired immunity.

Natural immunity is non-specific (it can act on many things), multidimensional (it works in multiple centers at the same time), and it has different processes that are both genetic and present from birth; for example, cows appear to have immunity to smallpox, but it can be fatal in humans (i.e., cows have a natural immunity). Innate, natural immunity is formed by the physical barrier of the skin and mucous membranes, certain chemicals in the blood, and special immune system cells that attack foreign substances. It is responsible for 99.9 percent of all immune activity and is our first and most important line of defense.

Acquired immunity is a later development in our evolution and has to be "learned" by the body. It initiates immune activity at a cellular level (in the production of antibodies) against invading substances and, as it is an induced response, is slower to become active than our natural immune response. However, once established, it creates a "memory" of the invading disease that prevents repeat infections from the particular antigen. So, continuing our smallpox example, milkmaids infected through their work with cowpox (a related but nonfatal form of smallpox) did not catch the deadly version of the disease because the body had already mounted a successful defense against the virus (i.e., they developed acquired immunity). In this scenario, the acquired immune system creates a secondary response to a disease, creating immunity either after a natural recovery or from vaccination. (Babies gain temporary acquired immunity—known as "passive immunity"—from antibodies in breast milk.)

In recent medical history it is our acquired immunity that has received most attention, even though it is responsible for only 0.1 percent of our total immune activity. The excitement and therapeutic potential generated by the discovery of vaccinations and antibiotics have dominated medical research and investment—understandably so, given how devastating some of these infectious diseases can be. But this one-dimensional approach has left our natural immunity largely untapped as a resource for healing. There is hope, however: like you and your immune system, the Ayurvedic approach to health is multidimensional and offers enormous scope for nourishing your natural immunity.

The integrated nature of the immune system

How you are feeling actually regulates your immune response. This is because the balance of hormones and the functioning of neurons are implicated in how the immune system responds to visiting foreign substances. Your brain and immune system are permanently communicating so that immune-mediated chemicals tell the brain what to do, and vice versa. Interestingly, studies have shown how different emotional states affect the immune system: loneliness reduces immunity and can lead to a higher viral count; excessive stress reduces immunity, and increases the risk of strokes, atherosclerosis (the thickening of the arteries by cholesterol), and high blood pressure, while reducing neuronal regeneration and accelerating the aging process. We know that carers of dementia patients suffer from reduced immunity, that people under extreme academic and work stress show reduced levels of lymphocyte (white blood cell) and interleukin (communication cell) production and have higher cortisol levels (a hormone affected by stress and influencing inflammation); bereavement reduces immunity, with reduced lymphocyte activity in men, and postbereavement depression can cause increased illness; marital conflict also affects immunity, raising blood pressure and cortisol levels, and reducing your acquired immune response.

But your immunity is more than what you eat, how you sleep, what you think, and how you feel. It's more than the amount of echinacea that you take. It's the whole caboodle: mind, body, and spirit. When we are stressed, our emotional, hormonal, and immune states "underperform," affecting digestion, sleep, and mood. The more we are fulfilled in all areas of our life, whether it is our work, our rest, or our relationships, the healthier our immunity will be. And the healthier our immunity, the more potential for happiness we have, and the happier we are the more fun we can have, and the more fun we have the better life is …

Symptoms of depressed immunity

You may be showing signs of reduced immunity if you suffer from any of the following:

- ❀ regular or persistent bacterial, fungal, viral, or parasitic infections
- ❀ slow-healing wounds
- ❀ autoimmune diseases, such as rheumatoid arthritis
- ❀ allergies
- ❀ inflammatory disorders, such as gastritis
- ❀ chronic fatigue
- ❀ depression
- ❀ chronic degenerative conditions, such as cancer, AIDS, tuberculosis
- ❀ feeling older than your age, with symptoms such as poor mobility, damaged skin, weak eyesight, more sensitive digestion

TRADITIONAL HERBAL MEDICINE AND MODERN ORTHODOX MEDICINE

Have you ever wondered why we have a modern health system that focuses on disease and the authority of the institution, rather than on health and the empowerment of the individual? Why is it a system that treats illness once it has occurred, instead of extensively promoting prevention in the first place, and where the rejuvenation of our health is no longer a priority? The answers can be found when comparing the worlds of modern orthodox medicine and traditional herbal medicine.

Modern orthodox medicine

Modern medicine is disease- and drug-based. It is termed "allopathic" because the treatment produces effects opposite to the symptoms. Typically it's what you'll encounter at the doctor's and in the hospital. Growing out of traditional healing systems, it has made some incredible discoveries and its advances in surgery, diagnosis, and health care have been miraculous. We know that, when used in the right way, its methods can be life-saving. Antibiotics, for example, can quickly remove the bacterial cause and symptoms of a disease. However, although the "magic bullet" of modern medicine can be very effective, especially in an emergency, it offers only a one-dimensional "cure." In short, its approach to healing is specific. And while this specificity can be very useful in certain circumstances, it also means that the medicine isn't able to treat different levels of complex diseases at the same time.

A pharmaceutical drug is usually a single chemical entity that acts on the body and forces it to do something: it targets one enzyme, one chemical pathway, one virus. In the context of treating some diseases this method isn't appropriate. Depression, for example, is often just treated with drugs that help the brain to retain more serotonin, a neurotransmitter associated with our mood and sleep. But depression is obviously caused by much more than just a lack of serotonin in the brain and so a prescription is not the whole answer.

Traditional herbal medicine

Traditional herbal medicine (THM) is the indigenous medicine of every culture around the world. As the name suggests, it primarily uses plants for their healing properties, but it also employs minerals, gemstones, vegetables and animal products, as well as techniques like counseling, massage, and meditation. Evidence of humans using plants as medicines dates back 60,000 years, but their use must go back to the dawn of time. However, we seem to have lost touch with this knowledge base – our great-grandmothers' generation was probably the last to know about the local plants that could help keep the family healthy.

One of the things that makes THM so effective is its assessment of the "lifeforce" of the individual. This is an analysis of the person's inherent essence and vitality, which in Ayurveda is called *prana* (*see* Nourishment, p.38). It's a bit like the *qi*, or "vital force," in the Chinese tradition that brings energy and warmth to our whole being. A healthy life force is the true meaning of health.

You would think that THM's capacity to treat our life force would be a bonus in any medical system. But, viewed through the lens of our pharmaceutical-based system, it has been recast as "bad science." The difficulty in measuring the life force mechanistically is at odds with "evidence-based" medicine, which needs to quantify outcomes in a simple and reductive manner. The problem with this approach is that we are complex beings and illness itself isn't always simple, either. Shouldn't medicine reflect this? Well, THM does. It promotes the integrity of the whole being, while using natural medicines that are often multidimensional and nonspecific (i.e., they work in many different organs and treat multiple mechanisms at the same time). Take ginger as an example; it works on your digestion, lungs, and circulation, while simultaneously helping to increase the uptake of nutrients, promote blood flow, and reduce inflammation. The strength of traditional medicine is that it uses treatments that recognize the diversity of our complex physiology. Because of this, there is none of the "one drug for one disease" approach so familiar in modern orthodox medicine.

THM treats the cause and the symptom. Instead of opposing the body's own functions, like many modern allopathic treatments, these healing methods encourage them—especially its life force. And, contrary to conventional belief, *prana* can be assessed. Ayurvedic practitioners do so by gauging the pulse, the brightness of the eyes, and digestive strength at every consultation.

Does traditional herbal medicine work?

It's an unfortunate fact of life that no medicine works all of the time. We are vulnerable: we fall over, we eat the wrong thing, we are born with certain tendencies that can be hard to fix. Every medical system is doing its best to help and some approaches are better at treating some conditions than others.

But what does "working" really mean? A medicine that truly works, in my view, effectively removes the causes and the symptoms of suffering and disease; improves health and vitality; is safe, with minimal or no side effects or risk of harm; is practical to use for the time it takes to be effective; is affordable for the individual and for society. So, in this context, THM does work when used in the right person, at the right time, and at the right dose. And this is not just my opinion: there are now hundreds of studies showing how clinically effective THM is.

According to this definition, many orthodox treatments do not really work. They fail to remove the cause, can be harmful in themselves, interact adversely with other drugs, and can be extremely expensive. While they are often useful for acute treatments or to alleviate some chronic symptoms, they do not usually initiate deep healing.

Are herbal medicines safe?

Simply put, herbal medicine is very safe. The World Health Organization collected data on 8,985 adverse reports from herbal medicines between 1968 and 1997 from 55 countries. This equates to 5.45 adverse reports per country per year. With 30 percent of the adult population in the UK having used herbal remedies at some point, this number is exceedingly low.

A 2006 report from the chair of the Coroners' Council in New Zealand stated that the risk of adverse events from herbal remedies is so small as to be of no consequence to legislators.

It's not quite the same when you look at the track record of pharmaceutical medicine. Pharmaceutical drugs and modern medical practices are now known to be the leading cause of death in the USA. A recent report estimated that around 784,000 deaths are caused annually in the USA from surgical errors, adverse drug reactions, medical errors, and infections due to hospitalization. For a more detailed discussion of industrially manufactured drugs and their side effects and effectiveness, *see* Nourishment, p.42-3 and Strength and Stillness, p.144.

Of course, saying "herbal" on the label doesn't automatically make it good for you. In this age of information, it's up to you to educate yourself about what is best for you. I would recommend finding a network of professionals who can guide you in making the right choices.

The integrated model of health care

Orthodox medicine is functional, mechanistic, and quantitative. THM is holistic, energetic, and qualitative. They both have a place. The difficulty is that orthodox medicine is promoted by government, medical regulators, and industry—in part because of commercial interests—to the detriment of our society's health. Additionally, our cultural values prioritize the external: that which can be "measured," "examined" and "controlled." Orthodox medicine is partly a cause, partly a product, of this ideology. It's ironic that the success of antibiotics has lulled us into believing we could attempt to dominate nature and disease rather than work with them. As a result, the more introspective, reflective, and individualized systems of healing have been disempowered.

For the majority of health problems, THM is an effective and safe first port of call. I often joke with my patients: "If you break your leg get to hospital, but for anything else, see a herbalist." And if you do need a stronger or combined intervention, then it's just around the corner.

IMMUNITY: THE AYURVEDIC VIEW

"Immunity is a strength within all of us that resists the causes of diseases and their aggressive tendencies."
CHAKRAPANNIDATTA, ELEVENTH-CENTURY AYURVEDIC DOCTOR

In Ayurveda, immunity is literally known as the "self-avoidance of disease." It rests a large part of the responsibility for your immunity on you. Ayurveda considers immunity in terms of both quantity and quality: how much of it you have as well as how effective it is. Its holistic view includes an understanding of both natural immunity and acquired immunity. This approach is like considering your immunity as a combination of the genetic bank balance you inherit from your ancestors, the savings deposits you make yourself, and the interest on your account.

From the Ayurvedic perspective, there are many components that build healthy immunity—*ojas* (*see* opposite), the heart, the eyes, digestive strength, and tissue health—and there are general principles we can all follow every day to achieve optimum health.

Constitutional expressions of immunity

Because Ayurveda perceives life as an expression of our potential, it is helpful to understand how our constitutional tendencies affect our immune response.

Vata Problems tend to appear when the person is depleted. *Vata* immune problems will manifest in lingering illnesses, chronic degeneration, wasting, and weakness, and requires immune stimulants and immune tonics. Tulsi and ashwagandha are good examples of herbs that help to nourish immunity and strengthen any *vata* weakness.

Pitta Problems appear when there is too much heat in the system. *Pitta* immune problems will manifest with inappropriate and extended inflammation, manifesting in conditions such as asthma, eczema, colitis, and Crohn's. Treatment requires slowing the inflammatory cascade and reordering the immune response. Andrographis and neem are good examples of herbs that can cool inflammation and boost *pitta* immunity.

Kapha Problems come with excess storage. *Kapha* immune responses manifest in abnormal growths and mucus secretions. This requires clearing treatments that reduce congestion and remove stagnation. Pippali and ginger are good examples of warming herbs that can clear damp congestion and strengthen *kapha*.

Your *ojas* and immunity

The quality of your genetic and acquired health reserves is known in Ayurveda as *ojas*. A difficult word to translate, *ojas* can be understood as the quality within us that nourishes and orders the functioning of the body and mind. In typical metaphorical style, Indian tradition says that just as ghee (clarified butter) is the most refined essence of milk, so *ojas* is said to be a combination of the most superfine essence of your genetic history, digested nutrition, and your life experience. As the ancient Ayurvedic text *Charaka Samhita* states, "It is *ojas* that keeps all living beings refreshed. There can be no life without *ojas* ... It constitutes the essence of your whole body."

If *ojas* is depleted, disease can set in. The Ayurvedic texts say that when *ojas* is low we become weak, tired, dehydrated, anxious, fearful, and that our experience of life becomes unbalanced. However, when kept at the right level, its beneficial nature is seen in the luster of the eyes, strength of the body, suppleness of the limbs, resistance to disease, efficient digestion, potent fertility, vital energy and lucidity of the mind. It is considered to be the seat of the life force (*prana*) and digestive fire (*agni*), helping to facilitate their roles in the body. *Ojas* sustains health, prolongs life, and provides strength. Its home is in your heart.

Just after I began to practice as a herbalist, a young woman came to see me with a long list of chronic problems: repeated infections, tiredness, early osteoporosis, and poor digestion. After years of raising a family, working hard, and not looking after herself, on top of some genetic challenges, her *ojas* was right down and her natural sparkle was dwindling. I was struck by how all of the above symptoms of immune depletion described by the Ayurvedic tradition stood out: with low confidence and lackluster skin, she was anxious, out of touch with her dietary needs, and was generally struggling in her life.

After a few months of concerted effort by her she came in refreshed and renewed. All she had done was follow a simple and delicious *vata* diet, take more rest, use massage, and boost her "overdrawn" health savings account with tonic herbs. Not all of her health problems had disappeared, but she was well on the way to replenishing the deep reserves that were the foundation of her vitality and happiness. She was back in touch with herself and she was healing. Her *ojas* was being successfully rejuvenated.

Your heart and immunity

Traditional medicine believes the heart is much more than just a physical organ: from the heart flow the channels of the life force (*prana*), the mind, and nutritional circulation. So, from the point of view of Ayurveda, the heart is not only the governing organ of blood circulation, it is also the seat of consciousness. We know that stress negatively affects the physical heart, but it also influences the immune system, which increases or decreases immune-related chemicals depending on our emotional state. Living with a sense of emotional balance is therefore an integral part of how we nourish immunity. Ayurveda's view of the immune system is borne out by its herbal remedies for the heart, many of which also have a long-standing traditional use for rebalancing emotions. I find this inspirational. Ashwagandha and amla are two great examples of plants that nourish *ojas*, tonify the heart, support you emotionally, and are beneficial for your immune system.

As we have seen, the seat of *ojas* is also in the heart, and it is said that from this wellspring *ojas* flows around the body to nourish all the tissues. So the "spring" itself benefits from regular purification and rejuvenation.

It is one of Ayurveda's gifts to humanity that it reminds us to care for our emotional as well as our physical nourishment. It encourages us to improve our own health by taking care of how we feel, gently nudging us in the direction of self-belief, while building a sense of inner peace. It is a priceless gift.

 ## Your eyes and immunity

Immunity is a response to our experience of the outer world and our eyes are said to be "the window to the world." Ayurveda states that our eyes absorb external experiences and feed directly into the heart. It is often easy to tell how someone is feeling by how clearly or brightly their eyes are shining.

Palming

Try this simple exercise as a quick three-minute relaxation to refresh your eyes and help yourself rejuvenate.

Simply rub the palms of your hands together until they become nice and warm. Close your eyes and place your palms over your eyelids, feeling the warmth radiate into your eyes. See the colors, feel the peace. Repeat as much as you like.

Many wise teachers have explored how using positive visualizations alongside herbs to nourish the eyes can play a part in supporting both rejuvenative practices and the immune system. Yoga includes special eye exercises to strengthen them and bring clarity. Certain foods are very good for the eyes: bilberry, blueberry, chrysanthemum flowers, amla, and triphala. Not surprisingly, they are also beneficial for your immune system, too.

Your digestion and immunity

A healthy digestion helps to feed the blood, which nourishes the heart and immunity. If your digestion is impaired then it cannot metabolize the appropriate nutrients, resulting in the depletion of *ojas*. If your digestive fire (*agni*) becomes impaired then toxic accumulations, or *ama* (*see* Cleansing, p.72), can clog your system, obstructing the nutritional and emotional absorption you need for good immunity.

> ## The nourishing essence of ghee
> "*Ghee is sweet in taste and cooling in energy, rejuvenating, good for the eyes and vision, kindles digestion, bestows luster and beauty, enhances memory and stamina, increases the intellect, promotes longevity, is an aphrodisiac and protects the body from various diseases.*"
> **BHAVAPRAKASHA**

Interestingly, 70 percent of your immune system is located in your digestive tract: the lymphatic tissue in our digestive system stores certain immune cells, which try to inactivate invading pathogens (germs) present in the food we eat. So, our digestion "talks" to our immune system.

The importance of good diet for immunity cannot be overemphasized: nutritional food protects health and prevents disease. The World Health Organization has shown that 30 percent of all cancers are diet-related and that 70 percent of these cancers are connected with diets that typically are high in animal fat and low in fruit, vegetables, and fiber. For more insights on how to care for your digestive health, *see* Nourishment, p.44.

Nourishing *ojas*

At the root of supporting our health is an understanding of how to nourish our essence, our *ojas*. Along with immunity it feeds happiness, fertility, and an appreciation of life. *Ojas* has sweet, heavy, cool, and unctuous properties and, because like increases like, it is enhanced by substances or experiences with similar attributes, such as ghee, oils, milk, nuts (especially almonds), honey, love, contentment, and calm.

Ojas is reduced by the qualities in nature that are dry, astringent, light, and hot. Hence, *ojas* can be depleted by excessive fasting, consumption of nonjuicy foods, too many spices, lots of bitter herbs, eating food tasting only of one flavor, pharmaceutical drugs, stimulant drugs, alcohol, smoking, exposure to the wind and sun, overwork, undernourishment, fever, infections, exercise, depression, sadness, irritability, anger, anxiety and stress. This is because too much of any of these removes the protective, juicy and grounding qualities of *ojas*. Some of the best herbs for building *ojas* are ashwagandha, shatavari, aloe vera juice, and amla (*see* The Pukka Pantry for more details on each).

YOUR HEART: THE HEARTH OF HEALTH

"The heart of creatures is the foundation of life, the Prince of all, the Sun of the microcosm, on which all vegetation does depend, from whence all vigor and strength does flow."
WILLIAM HARVEY, "DISCOVERER" OF THE CIRCULATORY SYSTEM

Ayurveda has a unique view of the heart as the source of breath, mental balance, and nutrition. This positions the heart at the center of both physical and emotional health. In Sanskrit the word for "heart" (*hridaya*) also means "the seat of feelings, sensations, and the soul; the seat of mental operations; true or divine knowledge." If the heart is out of balance it is easy to see how disease arises: anger is one of the highest indicators in heart disease and early death. In fact, regular outbursts of anger are a higher indicator in early death than smoking, high blood pressure, or high cholesterol. Depression is another emotion that increases the likelihood of death from heart disease. Not surprisingly, the success of any treatment can depend on your mental state: optimism has been shown to improve recovery from heart surgery, for example.

You may think of your heart as a collection of muscles pumping blood around your body, but the physical functions of the heart are also intimately related with our emotional balance. We even say someone can be suffering from "a broken heart." However, the heart is related to the mind not only as the center of love and compassion but also of discrimination, thought, and anxiety. What happens when a dog runs in front of your car? You are surprised and your heart rate rises. You are temporarily emotionally "destabilized" and your heart is affected.

Because your heart is the center of happiness and pleasure as well as the place of fear and anger, it needs to be nurtured physically, emotionally, and spiritually. To stay healthy, the hardworking heart muscle needs a continual supply of nutrients, oxygen, relaxation, exercise, pure liquids, and emotional nurturing. But when you are tense, your body needs more oxygen and this puts stress on your heart. If you are not satisfied with your life it puts stress on your heart. So, keeping your heart healthy requires attention to detail, ensuring that you have a good diet, are breathing properly, relaxing regularly, exercising adequately, drinking enough water, and are sufficiently loved. Although this seems fairly obvious, it's not something many of us think about often. Remember: your heart really is at the hearth of your health. It needs to be tended and nurtured like a good fire.

Heart disease and the use of statins

We all know that heart disease is a major cause of ill-health. Around two million people in the UK suffer from angina and over 1.4 million people over the age of 35 have had a heart attack. In fact, heart disease is the leading cause of death (and premature death) in the UK—one in five men and one in seven women die from it (94,000 per year)—and also in the US, where it accounts for about 25 percent of all deaths. Despite the gradual decline in death rates from all forms of heart disease, these numbers are unacceptably high for what is a largely preventable condition.

We have all been brought up to go to the doctor or pharmacy when we are ill and to trust implicitly that we will be given the best and most appropriate medicine available. However, with the increasing frequency of reports about the lack of efficacy or, worse, the negative effects of pharmaceutical drugs, should we still unquestionably accept what we are prescribed? The very nature of many pharmaceutical drugs means that they do not remove the cause of most ailments but focus on the symptoms (*see* p.106). Although this can sometimes be desirable (e.g., for pain relief), it is also helpful to have medicines that try to get to the root of the problem.

General symptoms of heart disease
If you have any of these symptoms, go and see your doctor and an Ayurvedic practitioner:
* tiredness
* lacking in energy
* chest pain
* "stuffy" chest
* difficulty in breathing
* shortness of breath
* water retention (especially swollen ankles)
* visible blood vessels on the face and chest
* poor circulation
* high blood pressure

There are many examples of drugs that do not tackle the cause of the illness, have questionable efficacy (and also generate huge profits), but perhaps the class of drugs known as statins is the most interesting. Statins are used to treat high cholesterol, which is considered to be the primary cause of heart disease. However, heart disease is a complex phenomenon that, from the Ayurvedic point of view, is linked (along with dietary and structural problems) with our overall emotional well-being and ability to relax. Not only are statins the leading pharmaceutical drug sold worldwide, with four brands generating over $20 billion every year, but there is an inherent problem with the way in which they are used. Drugs companies have "persuaded" people that high cholesterol is the primary cause of heart disease. This is simply not true. In fact, 50 percent of heart-attack patients have normal cholesterol levels.

If you think about it for a minute, it's not actually that surprising that high cholesterol is not in itself the cause of heart disease. Just consider the Inuits: their diet has one of the highest levels of fats but they have one of the lowest levels of heart disease. Statins (or HMG-CoA reductase inhibitors) encourage increased clearance of LDL (low density lipoprotein, which we think of as "lousy" cholesterol) from the blood by blocking the cholesterol-synthesizing pathway in the liver, and not by increasing HDL (high density lipoprotein, or "happy" cholesterol). LDL carries cholesterol to the arteries and HDL carries it back to the liver. While total cholesterol levels are important, the balance of HDL to total cholesterol is a better indicator of cholesterol health and cardiovascular disease risk (a ratio of 1:4 or better indicates good health).

The "cholesterol equals heart disease" theory is therefore dubious. If it were correct then it seems logical that a drug that reduces cholesterol would help people avoid heart disease. Sadly, this is not the case, although statins can prevent a secondary problem if you are at risk because of having already had a heart attack or a heart bypass.

Surprisingly, the occurrence of heart attacks and strokes is not so high as to merit such widespread use of statins, either. Heart attacks themselves affect only a small proportion of the population (1.6 percent of men) and the use of statins only insignificantly reduces attacks in those predisposed to heart disease (a reduction from 1.6 percent to 1.1 percent). In the case of strokes, 641 people need to take statins every day for five years to prevent just one of them from having a stroke. That's a direct cost of $1.58 per day per person per year for five years (a total of $1,848,323) to prevent one stroke. Therefore the NNT (numbers needed to treat, a measurement method for determining efficacy) is 641 to get benefit in one person. Along with not being very effective, statins can also cause severe side effects; the symptoms of muscle ache and weakness are common to many, while memory lost has been reported in some people.

Despite the positive marketing spin, some very recent studies show that men over 69 do not live longer, do not have fewer heart attacks, nor benefit in any other way from taking statins. Even more shocking is that women of any age appear to receive no benefit from taking statins whatsoever. By contrast, one in every three people taking statins will have some sort of side effect. The drive to reduce cholesterol in this way has also been shown to lead to a higher incidence of strokes, suicidal tendencies, depression, and other illnesses.

Nourishing your heart

Statins don't treat the cause of heart disease (because it is not caused solely by cholesterol), they can harm people and are expensive. We continue to take them because of a misplaced medical paradigm that focuses on "single-pathway" medicine rather than a complex systems approach. However, there are a number of excellent, tested methods of heart health that don't produce any side effects.

Your heart needs a regular supply of oxygen and must not be overstressed, physically or emotionally. If you are overweight or have high cholesterol, you need to follow a diet that increases foods that are high in soluble fiber, pectins and lecithin, and minimizes or avoids animal fats, fried food, dairy products, and salt. Soluble fiber is helpful for clearing lipids from the gut and encouraging gut flora to metabolize short-chain fatty acids (which can decrease cholesterol synthesis). Foods high in pectin can help remove cholesterol, while those that are lecithin-rich control fat metabolism and prevent it from accumulating in the arteries. Pollutants and smoking should be avoided, not just because they can contribute to your cholesterol levels, but also because they cause oxidation of your cholesterol, leading to atheromas (deposits in the artery walls) and blood clots.

Light aerobic exercise will aid weight loss, but can also help digest the common stresses of life. Unless you have a debilitating illness or are pregnant it is essential that you do 30 minutes of metabolic exercise four to seven times a week, to induce sweating. In particular, Ayurveda recommends nourishing yoga practices, such as the dynamic Sun Salutation (*surya namaskar*). Regular relaxation and daily breathing practices (*see* Strength and Stillness, pp.154 and 161) can keep everyday stress at bay. In order to combat emotional stagnation and develop awareness on a deeper level, practice meditation on a regular basis.

There are several Ayurvedic herbs that help support a healthy heart. Chywanaprash contains amla fruit, a potent antioxidant that nourishes and boosts heart strength. Arjuna is one of Ayurveda's specialist "pukka" herbs for reducing arterial congestion, lowering blood pressure, and strengthening the cardiac muscle. Turmeric reduces inflammation, balances cholesterol, and increases circulation. Ashwagandha helps reduce tension in the body and mind, as well as strengthening the heart muscle. Herbal teas containing chamomile, lavender, limeflower, rose, gotu kola, brahmi, valerian, oatstraw, and tulsi are good for calming your mind.

THE PROBLEM OF CANCER

So many of us are touched by cancer today. Both my mother and stepmother have had cancer, and my grandmother and grandfather had it, too. I see people with it every day in my clinic. And this is reflected in the global cancer crisis: one in three people in the EU are diagnosed with it before the age of 75; the incidence of most cancers has risen by 50 percent since 1950; and the current trend of fatalities from cancer is set to double by 2020 to a global total of ten million per year.

As an Ayurvedic practitioner and herbalist, I firmly believe that the prevalence of cancer today is because we, as a society, are taking the wrong approach to managing the condition. I don't have all the answers, but I would like to present some food for thought, which I hope will help you or anyone you know with cancer address the choices to be made with greater confidence and clarity. It is important to note that cancer is NOT a "self-help" disease. It is essential that you seek advice from qualified practitioners, knowledgeable about complementary and conventional cancer therapies, so that you are assured of the best treatment.

Causes of cancer

The causes of cancer are many: genetic, environmental, viral, immune, nutritional, and emotional. The World Health Organization (WHO) has declared that 30 per cent of all cancers are diet-related, 14 percent are caused by smoking, and 23 per cent by infectious diseases. As diet, lifestyle, and our immunity are largely within our control, this is very good news for the management of cancer. It means you can take charge of certain lifestyle factors, such as diet and exercise, which may both reduce the chance of developing cancer and increase the ability to treat it successfully. There are four areas which seem to be most implicated in causing cancer.

Increased sugar consumption Malignant tumors are dependent on glucose (the body's principal source of energy) for their survival. As hunter-gatherers we used to eat an estimated 4 pounds 8 ounces of sugar per year (as honey); in 1850 we ate 11 pounds of sugar; by 2004 this had sky-rocketed to 154 pounds 4 ounces per year. When we eat sugar our body secretes the hormone insulin, which helps glucose enter our cells to generate energy. The secretion of insulin is also accompanied by the release of insulin-like growth factor (IGF), which stimulates cell growth, making tissues grow faster. Insulin and IGF also encourage inflammation, a promoter of cancer (*see* below). If excessive amounts of sugar are consumed—or, as Ayurveda would put it, we eat more than we can digest—we increase the chance of proliferative cell growth, an essential factor in cancer's life cycle. It is no surprise, therefore, that cultures with the lowest sugar consumption have the lowest rates of cancer.

Chronic inflammation Inflammation is caused by multiple factors and it is one of the body's natural responses to healing injury or trauma. Wounds are rounded on by our blood platelets to stop bleeding and stimulate the production of an essential healing mechanism, platelet-derived growth factor (PDGF). PDGF sends a message to our immune system to alert the white blood cells, which themselves mobilize a cascade of repair molecules. These work together to increase blood flow to repair and regenerate the damaged tissue. At first, the inflammation caused by these responses is helpful, but if these mechanisms become chronic—and cancer works to ensure that it does—then perpetual cell growth ensues and cancer can be promoted. Ironically, one of our crucial repair mechanisms becomes a causative agent in the development of cancer.

Modern animal farming practices Due to a massive increase in consumption, farmers have had to look for more "efficient" ways of producing dairy and meat. Instead of the animals living off grass, as they did in the past, they are now largely reared in more easy-to-manage mass "battery" farms and fed a grain-based diet of corn, soy, and wheat. This has led to one serious imbalance in the animals' diet: the omega-3 to omega-6 essential fatty acid ratio. These fats should be in a ratio of 1:3 in our tissue. In grass they are in a 1:1 ratio, whereas in grains they are in a ratio of between 1:20 and 1:40. The omega fats work in a dynamic balance: omega-6 stores fats, coagulates the blood, and can promote inflammation (and the associated cell-growth); omega-3 fats help reduce fat, keep the blood from coagulating, nourish the nervous system, and control inflammation (and the associated cell-growth). Countries that eat the most (grain-fed) dairy and meat products have the highest rates of cancer—and by a long way.

Exposure to industrially produced chemicals As we have seen earlier, our exposure to manmade chemicals has dramatically increased over the last century (see Cleansing, p.80). The reason that herbicides, fungicides, pesticides, and household and beauty products are strongly suspected of causing cancer is that many of them are endocrine disruptor chemicals (EDCs—see Cleansing, p.81). Their shape resembles the chemical structure of hormones, which the hormone receptor then reads as a signal to initiate the function of that hormone. They are like a key that opens a lock. Estrogen, progesterone, and testosterone are all affected by EDCs. These chemicals all upregulate hormonal production, promote cell growth, and are fat-soluble. Their fat-solubility means that there is a tendency for them to accumulate as they progress up the food chain, resulting in exposure to concentrated amounts among omnivorous humans (and animals). This may also be why there is such a big increase of cancerous tumors found in areas that contain or are surrounded by a large percentage of fat, such as breast tissue, the prostate gland, the colon, brain, and lymph.

Dietary prevention of cancer

Changes need to be made to how we are living if we want the best chance of preventing cancer. These involve all of Ayurveda's core values: supporting digestion, a nourishing diet, regular cleansing, and rejuvenation of immunity.

The shift in nutritional habits over the last 60 years has had a negative impact on society's health: cancer rates in the same period have doubled (not to mention the sharp increases in heart disease, Alzheimer's, diabetes, and other chronic degenerative diseases). Of diet-related cancers, 70 percent are connected with eating patterns that are high in animal fat and low in fruit, vegetables, and fiber (WHO, 2003). We now eat 36 percent more meat than in 1950. Well-cooked meat, especially when barbecued, contains aromatic amines, known as PhIP, which are collectively associated with bowel, breast, and prostate cancer in human cell-line studies. The increase in meat consumption is directly correlated with an increased incidence of death from cancer, as evidenced by statistics that show New Zealand as having the highest meat consumption and the highest levels of colon cancer. Conversely, vegetarian diets are known to extend life and reduce degenerative diseases.

Other nutritional factors, such as high levels of obesity and low selenium levels in the diet, have clear links with some forms of cancer. In contrast to this, the increased use of protective oils containing omega-3 and omega-6 fatty acids is linked to a reduced rate of cancers. Phytochemicals (plant nutrients), such as anthocyanins (the purple pigment in blueberries), carotenoids (the orange in carrots), and polyphenols (found in green tea), have proved protective against prostate cancer. But with vegetable consumption dropping in the UK by 25 percent since 1950, we are not getting enough of these protective nutrients.

Nutrient-rich food protects health and prevents disease. This, together with your digestive strength, affects your specific ability to prevent and treat cancer. And the good news is that you can make a choice about the quality and quantity of what you eat. Read more about the best diet for you in Nourishment, p.64.

Using herbal remedies for cancer

Along with a good diet, an effective plan for preventing and reducing cancer should include a range of useful herbs. What is exceptional about the use of herbal medicines for cancer is that so many of them are what is called "nonspecific." That means that they manage a wide range of mechanisms at the same time and enhance the overall well-being of the whole system. As cancer is so multilayered, this "nonspecific" quality is a powerful tool for healing.

There are now hundreds of studies showing how plant medicines can effectively prevent and reduce cancer. Turmeric is a good example of a herb that, even in amounts you can get from your daily diet, protects cellular DNA from being damaged by environmental carcinogens and helps regulate inflammation. The Ayurvedic formula triphala is known to be toxic to tumor cells but life-enhancing to healthy cells. Gotu kola prevents tumors from growing and spreading by keeping cancer cells literally "in their place" and blocking their ability to generate their own blood supply. Andrographis enhances liver metabolism, thereby helping the removal of damaged cells from the body. Frankincense is famous for its ability to prevent cellular inflammation, which is a feature of cancer. Ashwagandha has been shown to offset some of the negative effects of both radio- and chemotherapy. Reishi mushroom helps to strengthen your immune response.

The best way to optimize the effects of surgery, chemo- or radiotherapy, or even recovering without the need for these treatments, is by using a specific and individualized treatment program put together by a qualified practitioner. At the heart of every Ayurvedic treatment program is the need to ensure that the person is nourished, tonified, and strong. I call it "building the core and nourishing the root." Certain herbs, known as "adaptogens," build this core by helping the body to normalize and adapt to stresses (*see* box, p.128). Their ability to perform multiple actions on a variety of organ and tissue systems is especially appropriate for managing cancer's multilayered and diverse life cycle.

Despite the alarming statistics, getting cancer not only takes a long time (the risk of developing cancer increases with age) but is also biologically much harder than you might expect (the body has many protection systems). However, if you do get cancer then you can draw on modern scientific insights, integrated with natural therapies, and target the life cycle of your particular disease. This is long and hard work, but I and many other traditional medicine practitioners have seen numerous people become healthier in their healing journey by using an integrated program involving many of the above solutions with (and sometimes without) conventional therapy.

THE BEST REJUVENATING HERBS

Ayurveda uses many herbs for rejuvenation. Often growing on the "edge" of the world, in jungles, mountains, and in extreme climates, these herbs help us "come back from the edge." Used properly, they improve our ability to tolerate stress, increase our immunity, regulate our hormones, enhance our adaptation to different mental and physical challenges, and make us stronger. In other words, they increase the quality and length of our lives. Here are some of my favorite ones from around the world. *See* The Pukka Pantry for more details.

Amla (*Emblica officinalis*) One of Ayurveda's primary rejuvenating herbs, amla is an adaptogen (*see* p.128) that benefits people who are stressed, need an antioxidant boost, have a weakened immune system, or are aging faster than they should. It is especially relevant when there is a history of heart disease in the family, and should usually be taken over a long period of time to thoroughly replenish. Amla is an ingredient of two of Ayurveda's most nourishing foods, triphala and chywanaprash.

Ashwagandha (*Withania somnifera*) The perfect herb for the twenty-first Century, ashwagandha has two vital benefits: core calmness and inner vitality. It allows us to adapt to the stresses of everyday living so that we are not wasting energy. This deeply nourishing herb gently rebuilds immunity and strength and slows aging. It is perfect for anxious *vata* types, particularly those who lose sleep through stress. Take it with warm almond milk to enhance its nourishing properties.

Chywanaprash This tonic jam is revered as an "elixir of life" in Ayurveda and has been used for at least two thousand years to rejuvenate the whole system. Its sweet and nourishing properties build the quality and quantity of the tissues, which contributes to the strength of our inherent immunity. More specifically, this unique blend of herbs is used to protect, repair, and tone the lungs, heart, and reproductive system.

Ginseng (*Panax ginseng*) Although not a traditional Ayurvedic plant, ginseng is one of the best rejuvenating herbs. It is perfect when *vata* is too high and there is depletion, tiredness, and weakness, but should only be used to complement a healthy lifestyle. It lifts energy, nourishes the heart, tonifies immunity, and reduces high blood sugar and cholesterol levels. Do not take if you have heat signs, such as thirst, headaches, and fevers.

Pippali (*Piper longum*) Part of the powerful trikatu formula, pippali (or long pepper) offers immune-stimulating properties. It is essential for rejuvenating the

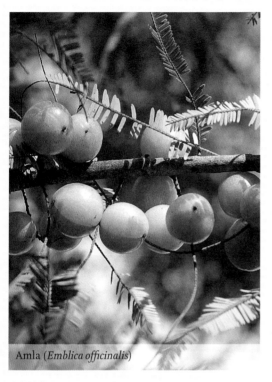

Amla (*Emblica officinalis*)

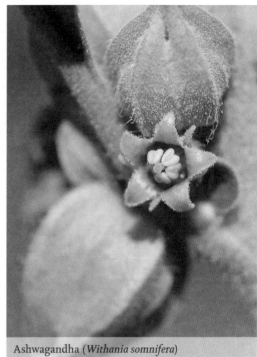

Ashwagandha (*Withania somnifera*)

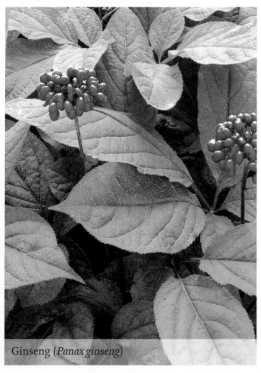

Ginseng (*Panax ginseng*)

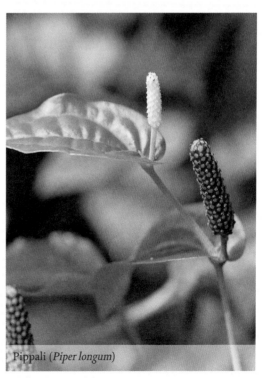

Pippali (*Piper longum*)

digestive system and lungs. It also has specific anti-amoebic and -giardial properties for the gut, along with an ability to clear *kapha* congestion and toxins. Using with honey balances some of its heat and directs the formula to the lungs.

Reishi (*Ganoderma lucidum*) The "mushroom of immortality" has gained fame for helping with compromised immunity due to cancer and chemotherapy treatments. But it's a great tonic to take when you are healthy, too. A superb energy boost, it is well known to help with fatigue and exhaustion and can be used to strengthen the heart and calm the nervous system. It helps to reduce the inflammation that can so easily challenge the immune response. Remarkably, it also reduces cholesterol. A full-spectrum product (one that includes the fruiting body and mycelium) will give the most benefit.

Shatavari (*Asparagus racemosus*) The sweet and bitter tastes of shatavari give it the perfect energetic qualities to reduce hot *pitta* and dry *vata*, while increasing wet *kapha*: cooling, moistening, heavy, building. These are often needed in women's health, and so shatavari's nourishing properties are used to rejuvenate the reproductive system, building the volume and quality of menstrual blood and assisting fertility. Although it has become famous for its benefits to women, shatavari also boosts men's fertility and heals digestion. Combine with almond milk, honey, and saffron for increased fertility, lactation, and energy benefits.

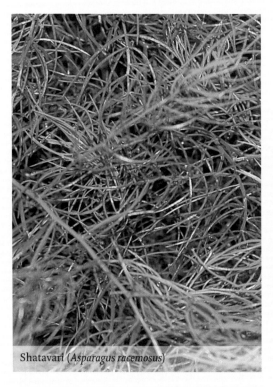
Shatavari (*Asparagus racemosus*)

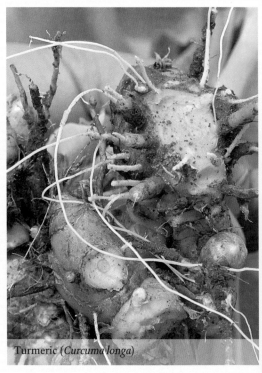
Turmeric (*Curcuma longa*)

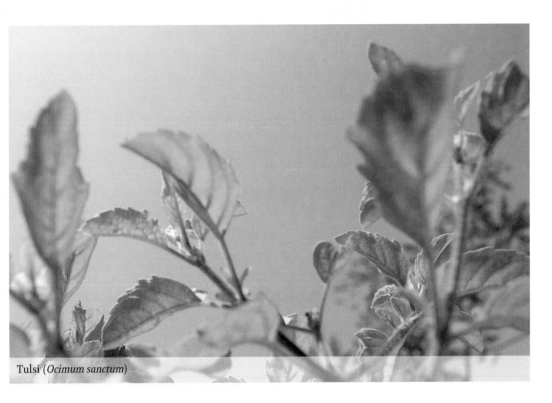
Tulsi (*Ocimum sanctum*)

Tulsi (*Ocimum sanctum*) This herb has an aromatic warmth that strengthens the body's defenses. Tulsi raises the spirits, lifts depression, and has anti-inflammatory benefits. I consider it my "cheat" herb for any chills, shivers, and aches with fever, as it induces a sweat, increases circulation, helps digest toxic *ama* and increases the digestive fire (*agni*). Drinking as a hot tea helps deal with early cold symptoms.

Turmeric (*Curcuma longa*) The "superspice" for anyone exposed to high amounts of pollutants and stress, turmeric prevents aging, improves circulation, reduces inflammation, heals wounds, and protects the liver and bowels. It has gained the reputation of being one of nature's most potent remedies for many age-related degenerative diseases, such as cancer, diabetes, Alzheimer's, and arthritis. Use it in your cooking every day or add to warm almond milk for a delicious golden drink.

REJUVENATION PRACTICES FOR LIFE

"While resting in the spirit, the mind, pure and stable, shines as a lamp shines with a bright flame from within the lantern."
CHARAKA SAMHITA

The renewal and replenishing of our health can be aided by the incorporation of certain practices into your daily life. Some require a more in-depth level of adjustment to your lifestyle than others, but all will pay dividends for your successful rejuvenation.

 Rejuvenation through the body

Moderate exercise (up to an hour per day) is known to improve immunity, but you should always exercise appropriately for your constitution (*see* Constitution, p.28). The benefits of regular yoga practice are invaluable to a healthy immune system. Yoga is a traditional system of physical, mental, and spiritual disciplines that is more than simply exercise: it is a way of living. Originating in India, yoga is associated with many of its religions and has become an integral part of Ayurvedic medicine. (For more on yoga, *see* Strength and Stillness, p.152.) Its practices encompass physical postures (*asanas*), breathing exercises (*pranayama*), and meditation (*dhyanam*). You don't really need clinical studies to prove its effectiveness (although there are many that have)—you just need to do it. Look in Resources (p.251) to find a practitioner near you.

Massage is a rejuvenative practice that should be undertaken regularly. Along with helping you to relax and feel energized, massage clears stagnant lymph and toxins and has been shown to improve immunity in patients suffering from chronic diseases. Massage also decreases the stress hormone cortisol and increases the "feel-good" hormone serotonin, so can reduce depression, pain, anxiety, and anger. *See* Strength and Stillness p.170 for further details.

Seasonal detoxification (*see* Cleansing, *Pukka Practice*, p.96) is a wonderful way to keep your tissues healthy.

Getting the correct amount of sleep is essential to good immunity. A hundred years ago we used to get an average of nine hours of sleep per night. Now the figure is about seven. This is an average sleep deficit of fourteen hours per week, 56 hours per month, and 672 hours per year. So, get more rest! This often means going to bed by 10–11pm.

Yoga exercises for rejuvenation

Practicing with a qualified yoga teacher will help you gain deeper understanding of the principles of yoga and derive greater physical and mental benefits. Anyone with a serious medical condition should seek the advice of a practitioner, as breathing practices strongly influence the nervous system.

Increasing the digestive fire (*agnisara kriya*) This is a simple and effective breathing practice that helps to kindle digestive fire (*agni*) and clear gas and constipation, while massaging the digestive organs and stimulating the appetite.

Sit in the hero pose (*vajrasana*): kneel with your buttocks resting on the insteps of your feet with your knees wide apart. Place your hands on your knees and, keeping the arms straight, lean forward. Open your mouth and stick your tongue out. Breathe in and out of your mouth like a panting dog. First expand and then contract your whole abdomen. Imagine a balloon is inflating and deflating within your belly and that each breath is fanning the digestive flames. Do five rounds of 25 breaths.

The corpse pose (*shavasana*) This is both the simplest and the hardest yoga posture of all: simple because you just have to lie down, hard as you have the opportunity to relax deeply, which is not always as straightforward as it sounds. This pose is excellent for rejuvenating your energy, removing tiredness, reducing blood pressure, and relaxing your body and mind.

Lie on your back on a comfortable floor or mat. Let your feet turn outward to relax the legs and open the pelvis. Allow your hands to roll over so that your palms face the sky and your shoulders are open. Now raise your head and check that your head, neck and spine are centrally aligned. Gently lower your head to the ground, slightly elongating your neck and let your eyes and mouth close.

Start to become aware of your breath flowing in and out of your nostrils. Allow your body to sink into the ground, becoming aware of all the points of contact between your body and the earth beneath you. Feel your body become heavy and your breath become deep. Scan your body and notice where you are holding tension; allow your breath to carry any tension away.

Practice this for as long as you like; five minutes or 30 deep breaths will help you feel renewed and refreshed.

Rejuvenation through the mind

There have been numerous studies to attest to the power of the mind in healing. We know that hopefulness improves the outcome of severe trauma and that emotional support speeds recovery from illness and surgery. Meditation has been shown to improve cellular immunity in geriatric patients. Relaxation and assertiveness training improves the efficacy of helper T-cells (lymphocytes) in men with HIV, and melanoma patients who learn stress management have improved natural killer-cell function and greater survival rates. Expressing your emotions (verbally or through writing) improves immune function, resulting in less sick leave, improved liver function, reduced asthma, and reduced arthritic pain. Dr. David Spiegel's groundbreaking work has shown how support groups have specifically helped to double the survival rates of women with metastatic breast cancer. *See* Selected Bibliography, p.248 for further reading.

> **The specific nature of adaptogens**
> Adaptogens help the body adjust to changing situations and are traditionally used to treat stress and anxiety. They:
> * reduce inflammation, regulate metabolism, balance the endocrine system, and check blood sugar levels and cholesterol ratios
> * reduce the stress response and inflammatory cortisol levels
> * correct cellular function, optimize protein synthesis and the function of all of your organs
> * support the production of antioxidant enzymes to protect cellular DNA from damage, which literally reverses the aging process and can prevent cancer
> * prevent opportunistic infections and enhance immunity in the face of allergies
> * increase our ability to tolerate a diverse range of pharmaceutical drugs
> * maximize the effectiveness of steroids, while reducing the associated short- and long-term side effects

To aid your mental well-being, try to create a pleasant environment. Surround yourself with music and visual stimulation —they may help to reduce levels of cortisol stress hormones. Lavender oil has been shown to improve mood in the workplace, as well as reducing aggressive behavior in hospital patients. Ylang ylang, rose otto, and frankincense are good mood-enhancers, too. Make peace with everyone around you. Have fun. A great Hindi adage says, *Sau rogon ka dawai, hason! Yeh hain mera bhai*, which means "There is medicine for 100 diseases, but laughter is my healing brother!"

Rejuvenation through the breath

Regular breathing exercises bring the lifeforce (*prana*) into the body and regulate the flow of vitality (*ojas*) around the entire system.

The Humming Bee Breath This is a truly beautiful rejuvenating exercise that will awaken your mind and nourish your soul. Sit straight in a comfortable position, hands resting in your lap. Take a deep breath and, as you exhale, hum like a bee. *Huummmmmmmmmmmmm*. While you are humming, bring your hands up past your belly, over your chest, and begin to caress the skin on your face, finally bringing your palms to rest over your ears, with your elbows out to the side. Let the soothing vibration of your humming fill your head, heart, and mind. When you have finished exhaling, let your hands settle in your lap, then repeat a few times. Be aware of your whole body–mind rejuvenation.

 # Rejuvenation through herbs

There are many Ayurvedic herbs which can be specifically used to aid rejuvenation. An amazing feature of most of them is their ability to help the body adapt to stress, which means they are known as "adaptogens" (*see* box, opposite). Part of their brilliance is that they perform multiple actions on diverse organ and tissue systems at the same time. Adaptogens also bring nutritive strength, are normalizing (i.e., they raise what is low and lower what is high, such as blood pressure) and are nontoxic when used at normal doses over extended periods of time. They usually have sweet, heavy, wet, nourishing, building, and tonifying qualities. Ideally, they will also possess the ability to revitalize the wellspring of health and vitality (*ojas*), replenish weakness in the body, increase the life force (*prana*), and kindle the digestive fire (*agni*). Adaptogens restore the body's innate immune response, which gives them preventative, protective, and curative functions against immune weaknesses. And the longer they are used, the more enduring their effect.

The wonderful qualities of chywanaprash

"*Chywanaprash is the foremost of all rejuvenatives (*rasayana*), especially good for alleviating cough and asthma; it nourishes the weak, the wounded, the old, and those that are of tender years as well ... From taking chywanaprash a person acquires intelligence, memory, attractiveness, freedom from disease, longevity, strength of the senses, great pleasure in the companionship with women, great increase in the strength of the digestive fire, improvement of the complexion, and the restoration of prana to its normal course.*"

CHARAKA SAMHITA

The origins of chywanaprash

Millions of teaspoons of chywanaprash are eaten everyday in India because of its revered rejuvenating powers. Its main ingredient is amla fruit, which is blended with around thirty-five other ingredients and cooked into a paste with honey, sesame oil, and jaggery (concentrated sugar-cane juice, which has unique nutritional properties). The story of Rishi Chywana, after whom it was named, inspires users to this day.

Chywana was a weak child, born prematurely, and was teased for being so puny. But he was never teased about his spiritual insights, which were evident from a young age. As was common in ancient India, his innate spiritual qualities determined his destiny to become a wandering monk (ascetic), and he left home at sixteen to seek spiritual enlightenment. His simple lifestyle further depleted his physical form, but he didn't mind: he was a monk and needed only to connect with the Great Spirit.

After many years of deep meditation in the Himalaya, he reached enlightenment at the age of eighty. His spirit was rich but his body had become old, his voice weak, and his energy poor. However, in one of his meditations he had a vision of the future in which he could bring more happiness to the world by living longer, contributing to society, and raising well-loved children. But how was he do this, with his body so weak and wretched? He began to pray to the Ashwin twins, the holders of *shakti*, the universal energy. Eventually they came, bringing a pot of herbal elixir. They said, "Rishi Chywana, because of your desire to serve humanity we have made you this rejuvenating elixir. It will bring you a strong body, good immunity, and potent sexuality."

One year later Rishi Chywana came down from the mountains a renewed man, married, and had a large family. The elixir became known as chywanaprash and its reputation, first mentioned in the seminal Ayurvedic text *Charaka Samhita* over two thousand years ago, remains unsurpassed.

CREATING A REJUVENATION PLAN

As health depends on many aspects, so does the treatment to restore it. A rejuvenation plan needs to be tailored to your individual circumstances and should target all facets of health: body, mind, spirit, emotions. I prescribe treatments that blend specific elements of these areas, depending on my patients' personal requirements and their energetic pattern. I try to touch the heart of my patients in some way, in order to help them ignite their own inner healing.

Treatment often includes various lifestyle recommendations. Internal remedies seem to "dredge" unprocessed emotions and bring them to the surface of consciousness, so addressing the psychological aspects of health can be worthwhile. Writing a personal journal facilitates free expression of undigested emotions, as may working with a psychotherapist or using specific meditation practices. I will also recommend "bodywork" techniques that may involve self-massage, professional Ayurvedic massage, yoga, or referral for acupuncture or craniosacral therapy. Incorporating a number of different healing modalities can provide a fully rounded healing process.

Diet is an essential tool for healing. Digestive fire (*agni*) can be boosted with ginger or other spices. Inulin-rich foods (e.g., Jerusalem artichokes and ladies fingers) and other prebiotics are especially helpful when the intestinal flora has been disturbed by antibiotics, nonsteroidal anti-inflammatory drugs, or just from a poor diet. When it is appropriate, I recommend fresh teas made with warming spices, or triphala powder or psyllium husks to restore digestive well-being. There is plenty of evidence about the poor nutritive levels in commonly available foods, so no matter how good someone's diet is, I also recommend a whole food multivitamin and -mineral supplement as a starting point for rebalancing health.

Our deeper immunity and *ojas* is nourished using chywanaprash and an individually formulated blend of the rejuvenating herbs mentioned earlier (*see* p.122). Medicinal mushrooms (reishi, shiitake, coriolus, or maitake) are useful for cases of extreme deficiency. Inflammation, so common in immune irregularities, is cooled using herbs such as turmeric, neem, andrographis, aloe vera juice, gotu kola, and guduchi. Burdock seed and root, nettles, red clover, chamomile, and celery seeds also work well. Calming the mind and soothing the heart are central to most treatments. I will often use variations of rose, ashwagandha, tulsi, arjuna, brahmi, gotu kola, licorice, lavender, oatstraw, and chamomile in the prescription. Herbal teas allow the actual colors, shapes, and patterns of the plants to be seen, smelt, and felt. A simple mix of licorice, green tea, and cinnamon works gentle wonders for immunity, *ojas,* and consciousness alike.

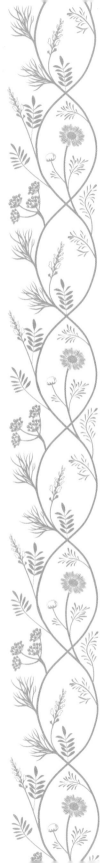

PUKKA PRACTICE

YOUR PERSONAL REJUVENATION PLAN

In order to ensure that you can regularly rejuvenate, you need to plan what you are going to do (and not do) and when. It just needs some simple thought so that you are organized and have created the right support for when you need it. Put some time aside to make sure that you can include some of these rejuvenating habits.

Daily living pattern

Body care Skin cleansing and self-massage
Exercise Yoga, walking, gardening, sport
Relaxation Breathing exercises and meditation practices
Creative outlets Music, singing, dancing, writing poetry or fiction
Emotional balancing Writing a journal, counseling

Healing treatments

Massage, acupuncture, craniosacral therapy, herbalism, Ayurvedic cleansing

Celebrations

Time with friends, time with yourself, mark special occasions with festive celebrations

Daily food

The foundations of a healthy immune system are based on a whole food diet. An important factor in sustaining immunity is the avoidance of poor-quality foods that have been refined, heavily processed, denatured, or are stale or rancid. Follow a primarily vegetarian diet that is constitutionally appropriate (*see* Nourishment, p.64) and aim for eight to ten portions of fruit and vegetables each day. All food should be organic.

The foods listed below constitute an immune-boosting diet packed with vitamins A, B, C, E, germanium, iodine, selenium, manganese, zinc, sulfur, and chlorophyll, and also cell-protecting flavonoids, beta-carotenes, antioxidants, omega-3/GLA oils, and prebiotic inulin.

Grains Millet and roasted buckwheat are alkaline and, along with soaked brown and basmati rice, barley, oats, quinoa, and amaranth, can mitigate the acidity associated with aging.

Beans Mung, aduki, chickpeas, and fermented soy products, such as tempeh, are sources of easily digestible protein.

Vegetables Carrots, squash, and pumpkin are high in antioxidants and beta-carotene; Jerusalem artichokes and chicory root are good sources of inulin; cooked alliums contain sulfur and inulin; the *Brassica* family are chlorophyll-rich anticancer agents, as well as being rejuvenating and detoxifying; also good are seaweeds, spinach, beet, celery, asparagus, globe artichokes, mushrooms (shiitake, oyster, maitake).

Fruits Eat primarily berries with skins, pomegranates, grapes, and citrus peels.

Dairy Only take dairy from grass-fed, organically reared animals; include some ghee in your diet.

Oils Use hemp seed and flaxseed oils, which provide omega-3; coconut oil is very good.

Nuts and seeds Almonds are low in saturated fat and contain vitamin E and phytochemicals, helping to protect against heart disease. Eat five, soaked and peeled, per day.

Meat and fish Stick to a vegetarian diet.

Herbs and spices Paprika (for beta-carotene), ginger, chives (for sulfur), turmeric, black pepper.

Sweeteners Avoid sugar and excessively sweetened foods.

Salt Keep intake to a minimum. Use sea and rock salt in your own cooking if necessary.

Superfoods Eat sprouted beans (chickpeas, mung, fenugreek, sunflower, pumpkin); microalgae (spirulina, chlorella) are good sources of omega-3, beta-carotene and chlorophyll.

Drinks Try green tea, ginger, fennel, peppermint, chamomile, cinnamon, nettle, licorice.

Daily supplementation

Take professional advice as to which supplements you are going to take, when, and for how long, to make sure they are right for you. Adjust with the seasons (*see* Ecology, p.197). The following chart outlines some typical examples.

Health routine	Recommended supplement
Daily tonic to protect and nourish your whole system.	Superfood "green" formula; chywanaprash; superfood phytonutrient formula (or something containing high levels of antioxidants)
Anti-inflammatory, antioxidant	Turmeric, aloe vera juice, natural vitamin C
Digestive tonic (before food)	Fresh grated ginger with lemon juice
Detox treatment (after food)	As required, e.g., triphala or fiber supplement
Nervous-system balancer	Tulsi for the mind; chamomile for the nervous system; brahmi for consciousness
Adaptogen and immune-system tonics	Reishi, ashwagandha, ginseng
Disease-specific formula	As required to correct any specific health imbalances; garlic, turmeric, green tea, and andrographis to increase the natural immune response
Nutritional supplement	Whole food multivitamin and mineral supplement

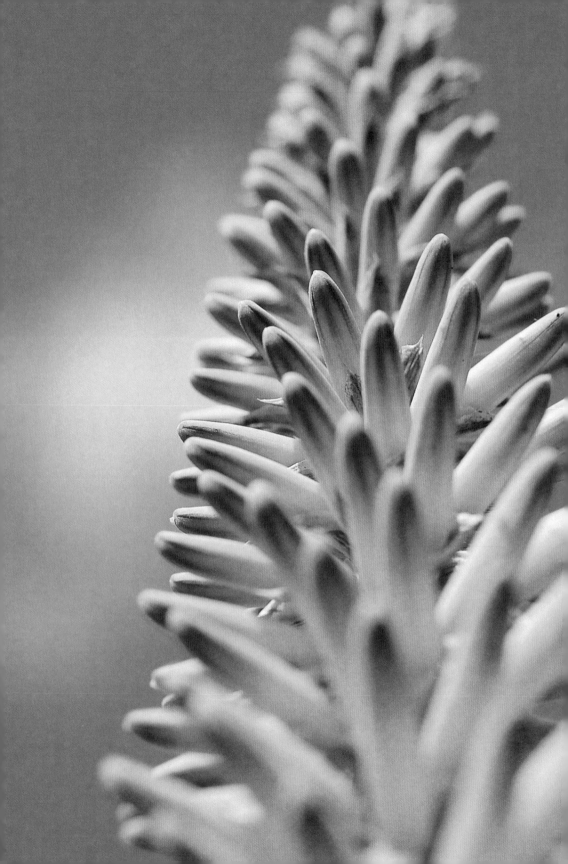

5 STRENGTH AND STILLNESS

"Peace comes when self is in harmony with the rhythm of the heart. This is accomplished in silent meditation by entering into the life-stream in the heart."

HAZRAT INAYAT KHAN,
FOUNDER OF THE SUFI ORDER IN THE WEST

Possessing strength and stillness is a sign of balance: power and serenity combined in one moment. It's challenging enough to hold either one, let alone both, in perfect equipoise, but that is the goal if we want to be balanced. Thinking of these attributes brings to mind resting in meditation, looking at a great mountain, or sitting on a throne. We can generate these "regal," even Himalayan, qualities and keep them in balance by learning to build strength and stillness through exercise, yoga practices, meditation, and looking within ourselves to the place of pain that can weaken our resolve and unsettle our inner peace. It may be a long journey, but it's a vital one.

THE AYURVEDIC VIEW OF STRESS

Our ideal physical and mental state is one of creative harmony but, unfortunately, it can be difficult to achieve. Before you can work on creating balance, you must first address the underlying causes of any stress in your life. None of us can escape a degree of stress, whether it is caused by external circumstances or by poor mental habits, but Ayurveda has deep insights into the nature of stress and what we can do about it. It sees stress as a disturbance of the nervous system, which is mainly regulated by the principle of *vata*. As discussed in Constitution (*see* p.15), *vata* has the natural qualities of being light, subtle, erratic, sensitive, and it is easily upset by too much sensory stimulation, too much food, too much time pressure, and too much to do.

Symptoms of stress

- Anxiety, being easily startled, and unable to relax
- Muscular tension, cramps
- Palpitations and spontaneous sweating
- Shallow or rapid breathing
- Difficulty in sleeping, insomnia
- Poor digestion
- Irritability, short temper

Today's busy lifestyle is all too conducive to stress, but there are some very good ways of being able to manage it yourself. As we practice how to relax consciously, we learn to observe our feelings and access a deeper awareness of the source of stress. In turn, we learn to find its opposite: inner peace. I cannot emphasize enough the importance of learning how to relax consciously. For me, it is an ongoing process, requiring regular attention to detail, humility, and a good sense of humor. I feel as though I falter every day; tetchiness, impatience, and a tendency to be overcritical are regular visitors to my usually happy mind. But, as children teach us, if we trip up we just have to get up, dust ourselves down, and start all over again—this time with fresh eyes and a greater understanding of what makes us fall.

THE AYURVEDIC MIND

Understanding the Ayurvedic concept of mind, and the body–mind connection, can shed light on some of the causes of stress as well as its cures. Not only does Ayurveda include ideas about how the mind functions but, as we saw in the last chapter, Rejuvenation, it also gives us an understanding that our consciousness is housed in our heart. As it says in the *Charaka Samhita*, "The heart is indispensable for normal mental and physical activities, as the entire waking consciousness rests there." From this we can see how attention should be paid to our emotional as well as mental well-being to be truly relaxed.

The true nature of the mind is brilliant awareness, and this awareness is created from many things: intellect, memory, self-awareness, ego, and consciousness—these become the content of our minds. A peculiarity of the nature of your mind is that, in contrast to your physical constitution (*dosha*) that is fixed from birth, it can be altered through discrimination and choice.

In Ayurveda, our intellect is known as *buddhi*; you can think of it as a mirror that recognizes your experiences and reflects the universal consciousness. *Buddhi* is the "digestive system" of our mind, discriminating between different aspects of our mental "nutrition." It is the "higher mind" that is at the very core of our being, responsible for determination, reason, and will. The penetrating and luminous aspects of fiery *pitta* that resides in the mind activate this reflective intellect.

The part of the mind that connects with the senses and coordinates thought and perception is called *manas*. It conceptualizes, analyses, and interacts with your inner subconscious, producing feelings and wishes, and orders your experience of the outer world, bringing you consciousness and awareness. *Manas* includes your memory and the ability to recall events. A common metaphor used to describe the relationship between *buddhi* and *manas* is one of a chariot: *manas* is the bridle and reins with which the intellect (*buddhi*, as the driver of the chariot) guides the horses of the senses.

The holding and storage aspects of steady *kapha* that reside in the mind give the ability to remember and recall names, events, smells, and so on. Your "I-maker," or ego, creates your identity of yourself. It personalizes every experience, so that you say to yourself, "I am short, tall, fat, beautiful, cool." It is our ego that says, "I am reading a book about Ayurveda." The mobile force of *vata* connects *buddhi* and *manas*, making up the totality of your mind. So, *vata* connects, *pitta* illuminates, and *kapha* stores our conscious experiences.

The three universal forces

Ayurveda understands that a further three subtle forces influence *buddhi* and *manas*. Just as the *dosha*s are the three great forces of existence on the physical plane, so there are the equivalent universal forces on the metaphysical plane: the three qualities, or *triguna*s. These comprise *sattva, rajas,* and *tamas.* The constitutional *dosha*s are held together in a balanced state of tension by the mind *triguna*s, which combine in variable proportions to create the mental expressions of *vata, pitta,* and *kapha.* They are present in every expression of the constitution.

Sattva This refers to qualities of balance, equality, stability. *Sattva* is light and luminous and holds the capacity for happiness. It is conscious and intelligent, moving inward and upward. Ascendancy, insight, and wisdom are all *sattvic* qualities. When you are full of love, openness, and calm you are full of *sattva.*

Rajas This *guna* generates activity, change and disturbance. It is mobile, dynamic, and excitable. It is the motivator and the expresser. It has a centrifugal force, causing dispersion and disintegration. This movement away from the center eventually causes the pain of entropy (disorder). When you are full of activity, energy, and passion you are full of *rajas.*

Tamas This is the immobile, still, and steady quality. It is heavy and, in excess, causes obstruction or lack of perception. It moves down and is eventually responsible for decomposition and degeneration. Through the force of *tamas* there is stillness and depth, but also delusion and confusion. When you are full of heaviness, stillness, and lethargy you are full of *tamas. Tamas* has the reputation of being a negative, downward-bearing energy. But to perceive it entirely negatively is to take it out of context and misinterpret its role. The fact that the *guna*s possess contradictory properties does not elevate any one quality over another.

The different qualities of the *triguna*s explain the variety in nature. The analogy of striking a match is sometimes used to describe them: the solid matchbox is likened to *tamas*, the dynamic movement of the match against the box is likened to *rajas*, and the light of the flame to *sattva*. They are all essential for creating light, but too much of any one quality confuses the nature of each.

The *triguna*s manifest in the quality of your mind and can be altered according to your lifestyle, diet, and mental attitudes. *Rajas* and *tamas* can accumulate and create agitated and degenerative forces—imbalances in these two qualities (passion and lethargy) are considered to be the main causes of mental disease. Often in my clinic I teach people how to balance these forces through breathing practices, meditation, and herbs to open awareness and regulate the nervous system. These are great tools for learning about the tendencies of your mind.

Constitutional tendencies of the mind

Each constitution, or *dosha*, has an inherent tendency to "think" and respond in a certain way. Understanding the qualities of your constitution can help you understand yourself and your relationships.

Vata Full of creative ideas, good at linking concepts, and communicating inspiration, *vata* people are also easily anxious, scatty, and are often seen as the classic "space cadet." They are quick to learn and easily forget—*vata* types cannot hold on to anything. They are predisposed to expect the worst, so the typical pessimist tends to be *vata*. Their irregular nature means that they often start new projects but become easily distracted. They oscillate between expending enormous amounts of energy on their social life and craving total solitude in order to recharge. They are sound- and word-orientated. Their emotional background is one of fear and *vata* people often have to face issues regarding security. *Sattva* is associated with *vata* because they both share the qualities of lightness, sensitivity, and insight.

Pitta Very intelligent and quick-thinking, the *pitta* mind is the collator of information. *Pitta* types are excellent at bringing information together and organizing their thoughts, and are primarily visual in their thought processes. They can be judgmental and critical in their outlook, are driven by ambition, and are determined to succeed. *Pitta* people are effective managers of anything: people, time, money. However, their inherent heat can bubble over into irritability and anger, though that will be soon forgotten (but not by *vata* or *kapha* types!). They are focused on their own development, which can make them intolerant of change and impatient with others. When imbalanced, *pitta* can manifest as anger, and they are often confronted with the challenge of patience. *Rajas* is associated with *pitta* because they share qualities of passion, dynamism, and heat.

Kapha With steady minds that can concentrate on a wide number of issues at a time, *kapha* people have excellent memories once the facts have been assimilated. They remember feelings, smells, and tastes. They like a stable and regular environment and are loyal and affectionate friends. *Kapha*'s love of stability makes them ignore signals for change. They tend to avoid challenging situations in order to maintain the status quo and protect their conservative nature. Their thought process is emotive and related to feeling. *Kapha* types have a tendency to greed and are often coping with issues of attachment. *Tamas* is associated with *kapha* because they are both expressions of stillness, stability, and solidity.

THE MIND AND DISEASE

"*From torment by threefold misery arises the inquiry into the means of terminating it.*"

SAMKHYA KARIKA

The mind is integrally connected with the cause and cure of disease because psychological experiences find expression within the body. In fact, your mental state is often, though not always, considered by Ayurveda to be one of the main causes of physical ill-health or imbalance. The term "psychosomatic" is often used when we say that a disease has a mental cause, but the word actually just describes how the mind can affect the body, rather than conveying the idea that the mind is the *sole* cause of disease. The correct term for mentally originating disease is, in fact, "psychogenic."

There is often discussion that a person's illness stems from "repression of their feelings." However, while the mind can play a significant role in some diseases, this is certainly not always the case. In any event, because everything is a part of the whole, nothing should be treated in isolation. The cause of disease is complex and often difficult to define; it is multidimensional, dependent on environment, genetic heredity, upbringing, *karma* (*see* below), diet, climate, relationships, occupation, lifestyle, prescription drug intake, and unique personality traits. Then there are external factors, such as divine, spiritual, existential, political, social, and cultural conditions. To single out any one factor as a cause would be a gross oversimplification and misrepresentation.

What is important in any healing is targeting the right level of disease: physical, emotional, mental, spiritual, gross, subtle. If it is primarily physical, it needs physical treatments, such as the use of natural antibacterials; if the disease is manifesting on an emotional level, then it needs emotional therapies, such as psychotherapy; mental disease requires techniques aimed at intervening in the patterns in the mind, such as visualizations or affirmations; spiritual level diseases require spiritual intervention, such as direct healing (e.g., the laying on of hands) or mantra repetition.

Alongside the timeless wisdom of Ayurveda lie many cultural idiosyncrasies, which attribute the occurrence of certain diseases to moral lapses. One such example is the notion of *karma*, postulating that a disease is caused by negative actions in a former life that must be atoned for in this life. However, I consider this to be far too simplistic. How does this help the person who is suffering? By them having to endure more guilt and social ostracism? The guilt and self-blame culture this view generates can itself be causative of disease and I cannot see how there is a benefit for the individual person in these situations.

Just consider this example. If you tell someone that their constipation is because they have repressed their feelings, all they will feel is guilt and disempowerment, as they do not know how to control the disease. If, however, you say that it is because they have unwittingly eaten an inappropriate meal, then they have control over what actions can be taken. You can then go on to address any psychological or emotional aspects of their health in tandem with the physical issues, and the patient is guilt-free and empowered. This is real healing.

Of course, the positive news is that, however disease originates, you can influence it with your mind: by being more consciously aware; practicing creative visualizations to see yourself in health; having cognitive behavior therapy to help you change negative habits; using affirmations to reinforce a positive outlook; regularly writing a journal to help you free your feelings; expressing your creativity so that your being is expressed in your doing; regularly entering into a state of mind so that you can give and receive love; and creating the space in your life to forgive, and/or having some practice to help evoke compassion for yourself and others. You can also influence your mind and any illness via the body through other techniques already mentioned: massage, your living environment, appropriate diet, and herbs. The spiritual-emotional practices of prayer are also important aspects of embracing total well-being for some people. The list could go on. And an important thing to remember is that just because illness causes us to change our habits it does not mean that the absence of these habits is the cause of disease. Adopting different habits is the cure. The cause, as we know, is often very complex.

The effects of stress

How deeply the mind and body are interconnected in disease and health is being explored by the fascinating scientific field of psychoneuroimmunology. The scientists specializing in this area are studying how our feelings, thoughts, nervous system, and immunity are interrelated. For example, studies have shown that when there is a surge of stress we release a barrage of hormones, which in turn leads to suppression of our immunity. This explains why people who suffer from chronic anxiety, depression, and tension are found to have double the risk of certain diseases such as asthma, arthritis, severe headaches, peptic ulcers, and heart disease. Strong emotions like anger are known to increase the risk of heart disease by decreasing the efficiency of the central nervous system on the capillaries and heart, and thus weakening the heart muscle. They also raise blood pressure and increase blood flow, which may cause micro-tears in the coronary artery where obstructive plaque can develop.

Even more concerning is that stress has been shown to compromise immune function to the extent that it can both cause and accelerate the spread of cancer, initiate inflammation, increase plaque formation leading to atherosclerosis and heart attacks, accelerate the onset of Type 1 and affect the progress of Type 2 diabetes, and exacerbate asthma and ulcerative colitis.

However, the opposite of the above is also true: decreasing stress by optimism, cheerfulness, and happiness leads to improved immunity, more vital health, and enhanced well-being. I am often heartened to think that what is important is not the fact that we get stressed but how quickly we can rediscover our calm inner center.

PAIN: A SOURCE OF STRENGTH

We all have pain in our lives. From the catastrophic loss of loved ones to the more subtle sadness of incessant change, pain is always with us. Much of it is unavoidable and we are often powerless to stop it. As a result, we become driven by our discomfort. Because of this pain we hurt and we suffer when we hold onto it. Certainly, we sometimes need to hold it, work it, understand it, before it can be known and cradled safely. But it still causes suffering.

The sources of pain

The experience of pain is a broad and complex subject, with different cultural and religious viewpoints. However, some pains are universal. They are the pains that fill the annals of our folklore and mythology, from Romeo and Juliet to the stories of the *Mahabharata* and Jesus Christ. Tales of struggle and survival have become the themes of our festivals, from Christmas through Diwali to Yom Kippur and Eid. These symbolic stories always relate to the fundamental truths of love, belonging, and wholeness. Every experience and myth can be traced back to the elements that run through all our lives: death, loss, illness, separation, and how to find eternal life, success, love, and integration.

Our response to pain

Sadness is a natural reaction to painful circumstances and a little of it can be healthy, as it helps us reflect on the realities of life. Sadness usually passes after a few weeks when you have come to terms with your troubles. Depression, however, has more symptoms than simply an unhappy mood and can manifest in a host of debilitating physical and mental challenges. It happens when we hold on to pain, without acknowledging it and letting it go. Continued feelings of unhappiness turn into hopelessness and pessimism. You become plagued with low self-esteem, worthlessness, and guilt. Activities that you normally enjoy, such as hobbies, work, or sex, hold

no interest for you. Maybe you feel sluggish and fatigued yet suffer from insomnia, wake early in the morning, or oversleep. You have difficulty concentrating and remembering things, and find it impossible to make decisions. Your overall mood is one of irritability, restlessness, anxiety, and even hostility.

Some experts say that chronic depression is caused by not being able to integrate our experiences within our lives. Many thought and behavior patterns start in childhood, before we can even speak or express freely. From the moment we are born we all start to tread the single path of how to find love, but the causes of chronic pain appear to be broad and varied: insecurity about being loved; learning an inappropriate reward-based system to receive appreciation; emotional, physical, or sexual abuse; threats of abuse; neglect; criticism; inappropriate expectations; maternal or paternal separation; conflict in the family; divorce; addictive behavior within the family; violence in the family; discrimination such as racism, sexism and poverty. If not somehow understood, digested, and healed, these experiences can lead to psychological problems that are then reinforced by learned social and cultural beliefs, making curative behavior difficult. The problem is exacerbated by the prevalent use of prescription drugs to treat anxiety and mental illness. Though often useful, they can act like a lid on a boiling pan of water; by suppressing the symptoms and masking the cause, the real roots of depression are rarely fully addressed and, consequently, often "bubble over," returning in habitual fashion.

The epidemic of depression

We are all aware of ecological, social, and emotional disasters and it's natural to be distressed by them. However, in order to "survive" we block them from our experience. Just watch the news or read a paper: we need to close parts of our emotional system to these horror stories in order to get on with daily existence. It's the same with our personal lives: we can't digest all of our experiences and so we put them to one side. But, if ignored for too long, this repression can lead to depression.

It is said that 33 percent of us living in the industrial world have some adverse psychological symptoms and that fifteen percent of us are clinically depressed, requiring medication and other forms of care. It's not easy on either gender, with more than twenty percent of women and twelve percent of men experiencing anxiety disorders. Over half of us have problems sleeping. In the US, four million people take antianxiety medications, such as Valium, every day. And it doesn't stop there. These individual sufferings are compounded by our social beliefs: 54 percent of people believe depression is a personal weakness; 41 percent of depressed women are too embarrassed to seek help; and fifteen percent of chronically depressed people will commit suicide.

Depression is predicted to be the second-largest killer after heart disease by 2020, and studies show that it is also a contributory factor in fatal coronary disease. Furthermore, depression results in more absenteeism than almost any other physical disorder and costs employers in the US more than $51 billion per year in lost working days and productivity—that's without including high medical and pharmaceutical bills. And these are big: 60 million prescriptions were written in the US at a cost of $10 billion. In the UK 3.5 million people received prescriptions for antidepressants in 2004, costing $472 million. One of the major problems with both antianxiety benzodiazepams and many antidepressants is addiction: 50 percent of people have some withdrawal symptoms when trying to come off antidepressants and find it difficult to stop taking them.

Adding to this worrying catalogue of statistics is a study from 2008, published in the *Public Library of Science Medicine* (a peer-reviewed, US open-access journal), which showed that a number of antidepressant drugs that attempt to increase the levels of serotonin in the brain (serotonin is one of the neurotransmitters that is associated with mood), such as Prozac, Seroxat, and Effexor, are linked to suicide, violence, psychosis, abnormal bleeding, and brain tumors, and were little more effective than a placebo for treating depression. But perhaps that's not surprising when you consider that our emotional patterns are dependent on rather more than just our serotonin levels. For deep healing we need to get to the source of the pain.

The point of pain

Many of the great wisdom traditions describe the inevitable nature of suffering and how to overcome it. The Buddha described life as suffering: impermanence, illness, old age, and death. We can't escape any of them, and in our efforts to do so we suffer. But though this sounds pessimistic the Buddha also offered the solutions to this suffering: to take refuge in oneself, develop compassion, and experience the emptiness and "non-real" nature of all life. Another of the great Indian philosophical traditions, *Samkhya*, also explains the nature and cause of suffering. Drawing on this philosophy, Ayurveda outlines "threefold misery": intrinsic (internally caused pain, such as our attachments), extrinsic (externally caused, such as natural calamities), divine (the will of God). Because we dislike feeling low, we investigate how to get rid of these three miseries—this, too, is the goal of Ayurveda. Christianity gave meaning to suffering by placing "unavoidable" negative experiences of suffering in a valuable spiritual context. It even perceives suffering as a means to purification and spiritual ascent.

Pain is a natural response to human existence. It's the price of being conscious in a world where challenges exist. To be awake is, on one level, to feel pain. But the pathology of pain is that when we suppress it and allow it to lodge in a defensive behavior pattern, it no longer serves us. Or it may live in a part of our body and disrupt our healthy physical responses. Then it is an illness. But pain has a purpose. It drives us to change things and to find a solution for it. The suffering pushes us, eventually, to take remedial action.

For all the types of pain that can lead to suffering there is a solution. Through opening our hearts with compassion to the pain that life brings, we can truly cure our pain and avoid our suffering. Then we can walk in the valley of love and experience the vast space within our heart.

ADDICTION

Addictions are rife today, with more people experiencing increasing numbers of them. We are creatures of habit; I have a whole heap of addictions. An addiction is one way to protect and bolster our ego so as to delay or avoid contact with our own inner pain. We use addictions to veil the reality that is behind them; by satisfying an immediate craving we put the "lid" on the emotion that is causing the craving. Looked at simply, we create thought patterns of "be good, get candies; be bad, candies withheld" and therefore, "candies equal love." And as we all want more love, we all want more "candies."

And from here it begins: from the "great separation" at birth, we journey on our path seeking an inner sense of unity and self-worth. Along with a plethora of idiosyncratic behavior traits, "drugs" (in their widest sense) help us to numb this painful feeling of separation, whether they be the seemingly innocuous TV, chocolate, and coffee, to more destabilizing opiates and alcohol.

We all want to be happy and free of pain and every culture has generated ways to get there. The very reason for the birth of Ayurveda was the alleviation of suffering, and at the heart of all spiritual traditions is the quest for the experience of the nature of reality, a quest for an eternal, unchanging unity, a quest for inner peace. The separation and duality that we feel every day is what leaves an emptiness, an undernourished part of ourselves.

We have to be open to find inner peace. Through following a "spiritual" practice and coming to understand the indivisible nature of our existence and our part in the interwoven web of life, the nature of our inner blissful and divine self can be realized. Until then, we rely on addictions and aversions, likes and dislikes, every moment of every day.

One thing that is guaranteed in life is that it will change. Hanging onto the idea that any happiness or any sadness will last forever is a common error that we all make. When a person can experience that life, good and bad, is all essentially the one same truth, then they are said to have gained self-realization (*moksa*). Any other focus or experience is an absorption with the transient, the noneternal, and the nontrue; hence, it is an addiction to the material world.

It is only through studying ourselves that things can change. Through self-enquiry, a healthy life regime, working in a field that is fulfilling, and living an ethical and virtuous life, all addictions, obvious or subtle, can be removed. As discussed earlier, Ayurveda is about choice. Any substance may well have a place for use at a given time by a given person at the appropriate dosage. For example, there is nothing "wrong" with tobacco *per se*; in fact, it is a healing plant when used in a certain manner – we just don't use it that way. Using substances that help us transcend our normal consciousness is a part of being human. We all do it. Whether it's alcohol, cannabis, food, or more modern drugs, we seem to love them. But, whatever our "tipple," the important question is how we do it and to what end. Does indulging in this way induce creativity, openness, and compassion? Or are you running yourself dry?

❈ Smoking

Vata types smoke as a nervous habit to calm their anxiety. They take quick and deep puffs, which actually increases stress due to the epinephrine released. *Pitta* types smoke to remain in control and enjoy the heat and fire associated with smoking. *Kapha* types smoke slowly and enjoy the stimulating effect of tobacco.

❈ Alcohol

Alcohol is used therapeutically in Ayurveda as a medicinal tonic for warming the body, giving courage, and calming *vata*. Quite a few Ayurvedic tonics are self-fermented to ensure preservation, making them herbal wines. However, in excess, alcohol damages the blood and liver, creating various symptoms such as a red face, poor digestion, diarrhea, weight gain, and lowered immunity. These are primarily, *pitta-kapha* imbalances, although in prolonged and excessive use alcohol will also aggravate *vata*. This is because it has directly opposing qualities to *ojas*, the vital essence (*see* Rejuvenation, p.111) which is sweet, cooling and nutritive. Alcoholism leads to "wasting," an illness known in Ayurveda as *rajayakshma*, or "king's disease," which is associated not only with tuberculosis but also with living a king's life of luxury and excess. Alcohol also contains sugar and its consumption may, in part, be a substitute for sugar addiction.

❈ Recreational drugs

Magic mushrooms, opium, LSD have all played a part in developing the creative, artistic, and spiritual aspects of our world. Whether it is drinking *bhang* (a cannabis drink) in celebration of Lord Shiva, taking mushroom tea in a Shamanic ritual, or sipping wine at Christmas, recreational drugs are a common part of our cultural milieu. However, any drug used excessively tends to damage the *sattvic* nature (*see* p.138) within a person, distorting mental clarity, and causing dullness and inertia (*tamas*).

Psychotropic hallucinogens (LSD, mescaline, psilocybin, DMT, ayahuasca)
These increase the mental fire (*pitta* and *rajas*), giving access to deeper realms of consciousness, but, when used in excess, they burn up or deplete *ojas*, thus making the person susceptible to immune-deficiency diseases.

Amphetamines These drugs scatter *vata*, weaken the nervous system, increase heat, and cause *pitta* to burn out. Amphetamines also aggravate dryness in the body, leaving *ojas* withered and depleted, which can result in conditions such as adrenal fatigue.

Cannabis Renowned for creating a deeper awareness of nature and sensitivity to one's inner nature, cannabis readily induces states of relaxation, bliss, and reverie. It moves *prana* (the life force) and increases *vata*, but in excess can actually induce stress. The newer forms of hybridized "skunk" are especially potent and aggravating to *vata*.

Cocaine This drug rapidly increases heat (especially detrimental to *pitta* types), scatters *prana*, weakens the heart, and disturbs digestion. It inflates the ego and distorts reality, and makes you very boring.

Ecstasy (MDMA) Renowned for opening emotional boundaries and creating a sense of open-hearted community, ecstasy creates similar imbalances to cocaine (*see* above).

Opiates (opium, heroin) Raw opium was once used as a very effective medicine, and its modern derivatives, morphine and codeine, are in use today as heavy-duty painkillers. In excess it aggravates all three *dosha*s, and disturbs sleep and digestion. "Street" forms of heroin are highly addictive, frequently leading to ill health and depleted *ojas*.

Coffee Although not strictly speaking a drug, coffee nevertheless has a similarly stimulating and addictive nature (frequent coffee drinkers can suffer from withdrawal headaches when they give it up). While it may be healthy on some levels as it is so high in flavonoids and certain minerals, coffee rapidly aggravates *vata* and *pitta*, as it is a burned bean that is hot, dispersing, and overstimulating. It creates too much heat in the liver, weakens the heart, stresses the adrenals, and can cause palpitations, dehydration, urination, diarrhea and insomnia.

✳ Food

Western society's sustained affluence has led to an abundance of food, which, coupled with poor nutritional quality, means that many people are overeating. When used to cover up any emotional "dis-ease," it becomes a form of addiction. In my clinical experience, it appears that most of us have some issue with food.

The whole mysterious web that is woven between food and our need for love can lead to some painful imbalances. A person who over- or undereats feels a lack of love or self-worth provoked by a sense of worthless emptiness. This may be translated into anxiety, anger, or oversentimentality, which can make a person eat or reject food to pacify their emotions. From the Ayurvedic point of view, overweight individuals may also be eating foods that are too "heavy" or "cold" for their digestive strength, causing *kapha* to accumulate. Undereating in turn seriously aggravates nervous *vata*, making deficient individuals even weaker. Both imbalances deplete the digestive fire (*agni*). Food addictions, because they are so close to the bone, need to be unpicked very gently. For more on food and the *dosha*s *see* the next page

Overcoming addictions

The best way to overcome an addiction is to get to know it, inside and out: what is the feeling behind the addiction; what makes you continue the habit; when do you do it? It is only when you know the root cause that you can make an informed choice about whether you want to continue with it. Replace it with a constructive habit using Ayurvedic, yogic, and psychotherapeutic techniques. Use simple supports that can help you get through the change you want to make. Lessen the cravings and withdrawal symptoms of the addiction through herbs (*see* p.168), massage, and counseling. Begin to embrace Ayurvedic wisdom in your daily life. Start with the practices that most appeal to you, like self-massage or a relaxation method, and then add more as you go on. Have patience, self-love, humor, and willpower—these are all great friends on the path to freedom. Remember to welcome them into your life and put yourself in situations where they can appear.

A healthy relationship with food

We all struggle to a greater or lesser degree with attachment to food, but a few pointers can help break any negative or addictive tendencies.

Vata Like everything about *vata* types, their weight varies. Reducing sugar is crucial to achieving successful treatment: while temporarily relaxing, sugar is scattering when taken in concentrated and excessive amounts. It can be replaced with nourishing nervine herbs for mental calm, such as ashwagandha, gotu kola, and brahmi. Mild use of whole cane sugars, jaggery, and raw honey are fine, but white refined sugar should be completely avoided. The best foods for grounding *vata* are complex carbohydrates: whole grains of wheat, basmati rice, oats; mung beans and starchy vegetables are also useful. Fennel, cardamom, and coriander are by nature sweet, which can help to stave off any cravings.

Pitta Although *pitta* types tend to have balanced weight, they can overeat spicy and greasy foods, which can cause heartburn and lead to weight gain. To cure heartburn cut out chile and alcohol; to reduce weight, avoid red meats, saltwater fish, greasy or oily foods, sugars, and pastries. Include fresh, sprouted salads, bitter herbs (aloe, neem, dandelion and turmeric), and chlorophyll (leafy green vegetables, spirulina, chlorella), along with barley, white basmati rice, and mung beans.

Kapha *Kapha* types tend to have the most "needy" relationship with food, which only adds to their innate tendency for storing energy and accumulating weight. Removing excess water and weight involves avoiding all sugars, salt, dairy, sweet fruits, breads (with yeast), pastries, meats, fish, and oily foods. It is best to eat between 10am and 6pm, when the digestive fire (*agni*) is most active. Hot spices help digest foods and boost metabolism. For sweet cravings it can be useful to take a herb called gurmar (*Gymnema sylvestre*), which literally means the "sugar destroyer." A pinch dropped on the tongue makes sugar taste like sand, which is a pretty good way to help break a sugar habit.

STRENGTH AND STILLNESS THROUGH THE BODY

"*The stillness in stillness is not the real stillness; only when there is stillness in movement does the universal rhythm manifest.*"
BRUCE LEE, MASTER OF KUNG FU

When the body is healthy and strong it is easier to gain insight into your mind. In Ayurveda this is achieved through diet, exercise, massage, and herbs, with particular attention paid to ideas of balance and the regulation of your own internal rhythms.

Homeostasis

Homeostatic balance is at the heart of our inner strength and stillness, and the practices of Ayurveda are like a shining light in this search for balance. Just as the nature of all biological systems is homeostasis, or a natural equilibrium, the Ayurvedic goal of health is described as the balance of the constitution, the tissues, the digestive system, and the bodily wastes. Life is all about regulation. When we fail to regulate we die. Both Ayurveda and modern physiology recognize that health is achieved through balance and regulation of the internal systems and structures. Ayurveda describes this regulation using the concepts of *vata*, *pitta,* and *kapha*, while modern medicine determines it through chemical pathways and feedback mechanisms that control homeostatic regulation (which corresponds to *vata*), metabolic turnover (*pitta*), and structural identity (*kapha*). In its simple categorization of the three *dosha*s, Ayurveda has defined the fundamental design of life and the design for health.

Exercise

Exercise is a great stress reliever and one of the best practices to improve health and strength. It increases circulation, improves oxygenation and the antioxidant response, builds muscle, reduces fat, assists with glucose metabolism, reduces blood pressure, improves digestion—the list goes on. However, it should be practiced in the right way, in the right amount, and at the right time—as with everything Ayurvedic, it is all about balance.

Vata types benefit most from calming and grounding exercise like gardening or walking; *pitta* types need cooling exercise like swimming or walking; running, hill walking, and competitive sports can be beneficial to *kapha* types, who need to be active (*see* Constitution, p.28). Practice so that your exercise program boosts your energy rather than depletes it. As the *Charaka Samhita* says, "A healthy person is endowed with strength, willpower, zest for life, and sharpness of their senses."

AYURVEDA AND YOGA

One of the best systems for helping us to deal with stress and find a way back to inner peace is yoga, which has had a long and interesting relationship with Ayurveda. From their Indian origins, yoga and Ayurveda have flourished around the world. They are as relevant today as they always have been; their benefits are as crucial as ever, offering spiritual insight, deeper wisdom, and stronger health. They are the perfect combination for enhancing our spiritual, mental, and physical health, and an understanding of the basics of both systems can lead to a more fulfilling life.

The six cleanses

The *Hatha Yoga Pradipika* (a twelfth-century yoga text) lists the six cleanses as: internal cleansing (*dhauti*), autoenemas (*basti*), nasal cleansing (*neti*), steady gazing (*trataka*), abdominal massage (*nauli*), and frontal brain cleansing (*kapalabhati*).

It is often assumed that yoga and Ayurveda have always been part of the same tradition. While in the broader sense this may be true, since they both developed in India, in a more specific sense they are two distinct traditions that have only come together in the last few hundred years. Of course, it is important to define what I mean when I say "yoga" and "Ayurveda." By yoga I mean Hatha yoga, the yoga of physical purity, strength, and mental clarity leading to spiritual insight, which is the most common form of yoga practiced in the West today. There are numerous modern schools of Hatha yoga, including Ashtanga, Shivananda, Satyananda (also known as the Bihar School of yoga), Iyengar, Kundalini, and Vinyasa Yoga. They all use variations on the theme of physical and mental exercises to develop good health and inner peace.

Yoga is really a tradition of mental and spiritual refinement, the art of joining your individual self (*atman*) with the universal self (*Brahman*). It rejects the first three goals of Hinduism (wealth, sensual pleasure, and religious duties) in preference to seeking the ultimate goal of life: spiritual emancipation (*moksa*). Whatever your goal with your yoga practice, it will certainly give you some tools to help you manage your stress levels.

Ayurveda, of course, also includes lifestyle advice, along with massage, diet, and herbal treatments. Its breadth ranges from simple daily routines to deep and sophisticated medical practice, all empowering the individual with greater potential for health.

The seeds of yoga and Ayurveda appear to have their origins in ancient Indian Vedic culture, but the direct connection between them does not become clear until the sixteenth century. Around this time we can see that they began to adopt aspects of each other's tradition. Yoga, after centuries of being interested solely in the mind and enlightenment, became fascinated with how this can be achieved through bodily health. Like Ayurveda, it began to focus on the "purification" of the body as part of its journey toward mental refinement, and so we see the introduction of the six cleanses (*shatkarma*) into regular yogic practice, as well as sensible dietary advice to help lead the yogi(ni) (male and female yoga practitioners) to liberation.

Ayurveda also adopted insights from yoga. It began to incorporate the tantric practice of using mineral substances (e.g., gold and silver) to optimize health and extend life. (Tantra is a vein within Indian religion that seeks to channel the divine energy expressed in every part of life to allow heightened awareness and, eventually, spiritual liberation.) It changed the yogic objectives from immortality to those of rejuvenation (*rasayana*) and virility (*vajikarana*), two of Ayurveda's primary therapeutic goals. The idea of rejuvenation became central to the Ayurvedic approach to life and is an extension of the yogic view that death can be kept at bay. Many Ayurveda centers and teachers today include yoga postures, breathing exercises, and meditations as part of their approach for reaching optimum physical and mental health.

Ayurveda and yoga are examples of the wonderful Indian trait of absorbing everything around them. They have added to and complemented each other and we are the fortunate trustees.

Hatha yoga and Ayurveda

The *Hatha Yoga Pradipika* is a seminal work on Hatha yoga that represents the contemporary approach to spiritual liberation, using physical, breathing, and meditative techniques. It shows how yoga has absorbed some of Ayurveda's core principles.

"*When fat or mucus is excessive then the six cleansing procedures* (shatkarma) *should be practiced before pranayama. Others in whom the doshas are balanced should not do them.*"
HATHA YOGA PRADIPIKA 2.21.

"*Abdominal churning* (nauli) *is the foremost of the Hatha yoga practices. It kindles the digestive fire, removing indigestion, sluggish digestion, and all disorders of the doshas and brings about happiness.*"
HATHA YOGA PRADIPIKA 2.34.

"*Perform exhalation and inhalation rapidly like the bellows (of a blacksmith). This is called* kapalabhati *and it destroys all mucus disorders.*"
HATHA YOGA PRADIPIKA 2.35.

"*Sun pranayama* (surybheda) *is excellent for purifying the cranium and destroying imbalances of the wind dosha and eliminates worms.*"
HATHA YOGA PRADIPIKA 2.50.

Strength and Stillness 153

RELAXATION ROUTINES

An essential part of your health regime is the incorporation of relaxation practices. Even setting aside just a few minutes each morning and evening for some yoga, or taking a break at some point in the day for a breathing exercise, will bring you many health benefits.

Relaxation through the body

Most exercise is relaxing to some degree, but yoga is particularly beneficial. All inverted poses, twists, and backward bends help to relieve *vata* and settle the nervous system. Think about regulating and grounding *vata* when trying to relax. The following yoga postures work especially well.

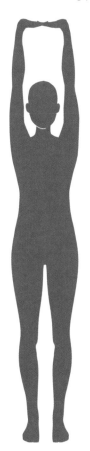

The wind-relieving pose (*pawan muktasana*) This simple yet profound exercise frees (*mukt*) any blockages caused by wind (*pawan*, the same as *vata*) occurring in the joints, bringing renewed energy to your body and mind. When *vata* that is lodged in a joint is freed you can hear your joints "crack." To help keep the energy flowing in your body and mind simply flex or rotate your toes, ankles, knees, hips, fingers, elbows, shoulders, and neck, in that order, using slow and thoughtful movements. Following your breath, rotate or move each of these "junctions" five times in each direction to free any stagnation.

Heavenly stretch (*tadasana*) Stand with your feet hip-width apart and interlock your fingers with the palms facing upward. Breathe out and soften your body. As you start to breathe in, straighten your arms and slowly start to raise your hands, rotating them outward at the heart. Push the palms toward the sky as you rise onto tiptoes, just as your breath fills your lungs. Hold for a few seconds and then start to exhale as you lower your arms and come back onto your heels. Tilt the pelvis toward the navel, tucking the buttocks under, and bend your knees. Have a few breaths and repeat.

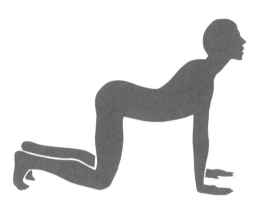

The cat (*marjarasana*) Kneel on all fours in a tabletop position, with your weight evenly spread between your knees and hands, toes tucked under your feet and your head hanging loosely down. Wiggle your bottom and let your hips and pelvis settle. Take a deep breath in and very gently lower your navel toward the floor, arching your back into a concave bowl-like shape, raising your head and pushing the base of your spine away from your head. Hold for a second. Now start to breath out, releasing any tension, and move your belly button up toward the ceiling to make your back round. Tuck the base of your spine under your pelvis and bring your chin to your chest. Hold for a second.

Repeat this five times, moving gently and with awareness. Then settle back onto your heels and rest your head on the floor in front of your knees.

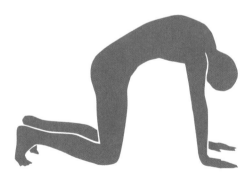

YOGA FOR THE *DOSHAS*

For each constitutional type there are a number of postures that are of particular benefit, although anyone can practice them if they have specific symptoms that need addressing. These are best undertaken by those with some experience of yoga, or in a class, or with a teacher (*see* Resources p.251 for further details), so specific instructions have not been supplied.

Postures for *vata*: to help ground, strengthen, and center

These postures are warming, stretching, and calming, and should be practiced slowly and synchronized with slow breathing. Emphasis is on connecting the whole body, slowing it down and fostering inner strength to reduce *vata*, create warmth, and settle digestion.

Wind-relieving pose (*pawan muktasana*) Joint rotation sequence to clear *vata* from the joints
Sun Salutation (*surya namaskar*) Slowly, three to six rounds, with deep breathing
Corpse pose (*shavasana*) Frequently, in between postures, for grounding
Heavenly Stretch (*tadasana*) Moves *vata* throughout the system (*see* p.154)

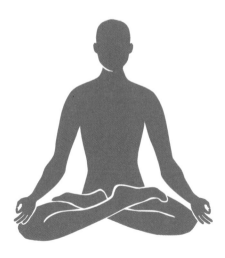

Moon pose (*shashankasana*) Grounds *vata*
Camel pose (*ushtrasana*) and **Cat pose** (*marjarasana—see* p.155) Backward bends open out contraction in the spine and abdomen
Lotus pose (*padmasana*) or **Accomplished pose (*siddhasana*)** Good for meditation
Tailor pose (*baddha konasana*) Opens the pelvis
Headstand (*shirshasana*) and **Shoulder Stand (*sarvangasana*)** Inverted postures help to balance *vata* by moving energy in the body
Eagle pose (*garudasana*) and **Dancing Shiva's pose (*natarajasana*)** Balancing postures regulate the nervous system

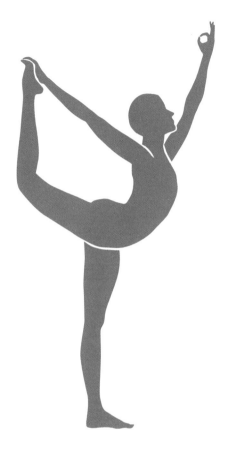

Postures for *pitta*: to help cool, regulate, and balance

These postures are cooling, stretching, and relaxing, and should be practiced at a medium pace and synchronized with slow breathing. Emphasis is on stretching the sides of the body, toning the liver, and massaging the abdomen to help regulate *pitta* and clear heat.

Moon Salutation (*chandra namaskar*) Slowly, nine rounds, cooling
Sun Salutation (*surya namaskar*) Medium pace, nine rounds, regulating
Half Spinal Twist (*ardha matsyendrasana*) Tones the liver and pancreas
Shoulder Stand (*sarvangasana*) Regulates the endocrine system
Plough pose (*halasana*) Regulates the endocrine system
Bow pose (*dhanurasana*) Massages the abdomen

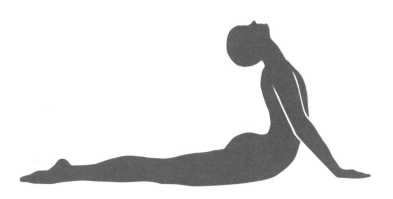

Cobra pose (*bhujangasana*) Massages the abdomen
Fish pose (*matsyasana*) Stretches the abdomen
Triangle pose (*trikonasana*) and **Slanting Mountain pose (*tiryaka tadasana*)**
Sideways bends tone the liver
Peacock pose (*mayurasana*) Massages the abdomen and stimulates the liver
Eye-gazing exercises (*trataka—see* p.166) Relieves *pitta* from the eyes
Accomplished pose (*siddhasana*) Good for meditation

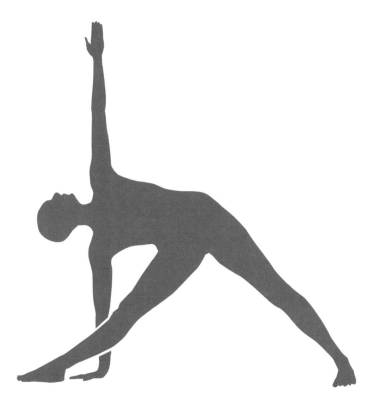

Postures for *kapha*: to help warm, stimulate, and invigorate

These postures are warming, invigorating, and powerful, and should be practiced at a fast pace and synchronized with deep breathing. Emphasis is on the lower back, the lungs, and stimulating the abdomen to help regulate *kapha* and clear sluggishness.

Sun Salutation (*surya namaskar*) Fast, twelve rounds, increases metabolism
Forward Stretch (*pashchimottanasana*) Opens the spine and nourishes the kidneys
Camel pose (*ushtrasana*) and **Cat pose (*marjarasana—see* p.155)** Backbends tonify the kidneys and open the lungs
Locust pose (*shalabhasana*) Tonifies the kidneys
Shoulder Stand (*sarvangasana*) Helps regulate the thyroid
Wheel pose (*chakrasana*) Opens the lungs
Peacock pose (*mayurasana*) Stimulates digestion and clears *kapha*
Cow pose (*gomukhasana*) Opens the chest
Tiger pose (*simhasana*) Clears the lungs, brings strength, and is good for meditation

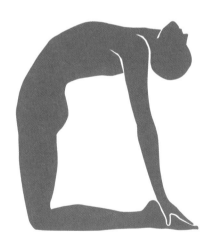

The making of a yogi

The story of Dattatreya, the original yogi, is an example of how important it is for those who practice yoga to keep their mind clear by being free from stress, practicing postures regularly, and contemplating truth. It is only by knowing Truth that the yogi can live in Truth, despite how it may appear from the outside.

Dattatreya was a gift to his parents from the gods Brahma, Vishnu, and Shiva, who decided to blend their respective powers of creation, preservation, and destruction together with the embodiment of the Universal Spirit. Dattatreya became an ascetic, renouncing the world. His approach, however, was unconventional: he took to wine, womanizing, and song, knowing that these pleasures were merely transitory. He learned that during the journey of experiencing the soul different temptations distract the mind and draw you outside yourself. His journey taught him the truth: that your essence is within, not outside. A yogi can experience everything, and yet still keep his gaze on the inner light. They can live in the world and still live with the Spirit.

Dattatreya taught that the foundation of yoga was internal wisdom: understanding one's senses, embodying simplicity, and emanating nonviolence. A yogi must practice meditation in a peaceful place, especially in nature. An accomplished yogi has control over his speech, thoughts, and action. Iron and gold have equal worth in a yogi's eye; he loves no one and hates no one. Dattatreya taught that chanting "Om" leads to inner wisdom —"A," "U" and "M," are the three syllables embodied in that sound, representing the virtues of *sattva, rajas,* and *tamas*: light, dynamism, and stillness.

A yogi understands that attachment is the cause of both sorrow and happiness. Being caught up with our experiences of life is what causes problems. A small sprout of self-importance ultimately develops into a huge tree of misunderstandings. Attraction is the trunk of this tree. Our family are the branches and our lifestyle is the leaves. Food and fulfillment are the flowers. Happiness and sorrow are the fruits. Our relationship with these experiences is the canopy of the tree. If we are too averse or overly attached to anything, the canopy will grow and obstruct the light that helps us to see our way to inner peace. So, we need to keep perspective. Celebrate your successes, honor your losses, and, like the spectral leaves of fall, let them float to the ground. Then you are free. Then you are a yogi.

STRENGTH AND STILLNESS THROUGH THE BREATH

"*Within you there is a stillness and a sanctuary to which you can retreat at any time and be yourself.*"

HERMANN HESSE, LITERARY MYSTIC

The yogic practice of conscious control of the breath is called *pranayama*. Its benefits are simply described in *Hatha Yoga Pradipika* (*Light on Yoga*): "By proper practice of *pranayama* all diseases are eradicated … The breath should be skillfully inhaled, exhaled, and retained so that perfection is retained." While this goal of perfection might take some time to reach, the benefits of serious practice are immediate. Proper breathing helps us to feel more relaxed, more connected and allows us to tap into the wellspring of our innate energy reserves. We breathe all the time, around 250 million times in our lifetime, but we are so rarely aware of our breath's ebb and flow. Our breathing is mostly unconscious, perpetually managed by the respiratory center in the brain, but, unlike other unconscious functions such as regulating body temperature and metabolism, we can control it.

The higher brain center in the cerebral cortex can take control of our breath just by our thinking about changing the depth, rate, and pattern of breathing. And the effects of doing this can bring profound benefits to your mood, creativity, and life. There are numerous practices to help us master our breathing, such as "alternate nostril breathing" (*nadi shodhana—see* the next page) or just simple "breath awareness" (*prana vidya—see* p.166) and it is best to start with one of these simple practices. To learn some of the more complex breathing exercises, try and find a good teacher to help guide you through the subtleties of this ancient art.

Basic breathing practice

Sit comfortably in a chair with your feet firmly on the floor. Make sure your spine is straight and you feel comfortable to sit in this position for about ten minutes.

Close your eyes. Start to notice how you feel: are you hot or cold? Is any part of your body tense? Move your awareness from your toes, up your legs, up through the back until you reach the top of your head. Then bring your attention down through the face, noticing any tension in between your eyebrows, around your eyes, or in your jaw. Let it all go.

Now bring your awareness to your belly and to how you are breathing: is your breath deep or shallow, fast or slow, long or short? Nothing is right or wrong; just observe how you are breathing naturally.

Slowly begin to take control of your breath. Breathe deeply into your belly. You should feel your tummy expand and contract, up and down, in and out.

When you have done five belly breaths, allow your breath to expand up to your chest. Firstly fill up your belly and then your chest, then exhale from the chest and then from the belly. It is like a wave flowing in and flowing out. Visualize this wave rolling in and out. Do this ten times.

Now let your normal breath return. Notice how you are feeling, feel your feet on the floor and the weight of your body on the chair. Slowly open your eyes and come back to the present.

✳ The victory breath *(ujjayi pranayama)*
Follow the same procedure as outlined above, but this time slow your breathing down still further while at the same time contracting the glottis. To do this, tighten the back of your throat so that you can feel a mild pressure in your nasal passages. When you breathe you can hear a subtle sound inside your head, rather like when you put a seashell over your ear. This deep-breathing exercise calms your mind and sends you into a profound sense of bliss.

✳ Alternate nostril breathing (*nadi shodhana*)
This can be a very purifying practice and is deliciously calming. It involves controlling the flow of the breath through each nostril in turn. Sit in a comfortable position (cross-legged on the floor or in a chair). Rest your right thumb next to your right nostril, place your index and middle finger on your eyebrow-center (your "third eye") and then hold your ring finger next to your left nostril. Your right elbow should be down in front of your chest and your shoulders should be relaxed. Your left hand can rest on your left knee.

To start, close the right nostril with your right thumb and inhale slowly through the left nostril while counting up to five. Then close the left nostril with your ring finger and at the same time remove your thumb from the right nostril, and exhale through this nostril while counting up to five. This completes half a round.

Inhale through the right nostril for five seconds then close the right nostril with your right thumb and exhale through the left nostril for five seconds. This completes one full round. Try and do five to ten rounds. There are many variations regarding the counting that are best learned with an experienced yoga practitioner (*see* Resources, p.251).

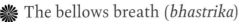

The bellows breath (*bhastrika*)

This invigorates your whole system, strengthening digestion, the lungs, and your mind. It involves consciously and rhythmically breathing in and expanding the belly and then breathing out forcefully while contracting the belly, like the opening and closing of a pair of bellows used to fan a fire. It differs from the brain-cleansing breath (*kapalabhati—see* Cleansing, p.88) in that the breath is exaggerated on both the in and the out breath, not just on the out breath. If you have high or low blood pressure, glaucoma, or a hernia this practice should not be undertaken without the guidance of an experienced yoga teacher.

Sit in comfortable cross-legged position. Either rest your hands on your knees, palms up and with your index finger and thumb touching, or interlink your hands over your belly button to feel the breath flowing in and out. Soften your whole body. Tune into your natural breath, the smooth flow of life, in and out. When you are ready, breathe in deeply. As you inhale let your belly expand. The lungs will be filled with air as the diaphragm is forced downward and draws the lungs down.

Exhale by firmly contracting your abdominal muscles and forcing the air from your lungs. Your diaphragm will contract, reducing the space in the abdominal cavity and pushing the stale air from your lungs. You can hear a soft "rushing" sound from your nostrils. Allow yourself to inhale, then exhale. Breathing in, full belly, breathing out, empty belly. Repeat.

Start with ten repetitions and increase by five per day as you feel comfortable. It is important to remember to keep your upper body still during the practice. It's an incredibly strong breath, and some people can feel a bit dizzy; if you do, just take it more slowly.

> "Bhastrika *quickly arouses* kundalini. *It is pleasant and beneficial, and removes obstruction due to excess mucus* (kapha) *accumulated at the entrance to* brahma nadi ... *This enables the three psychic knots to be broken. Thus it is the duty of the yogi to practice* bhastrika."
> ***HATHA YOGA PRADIPIKA***

Kundalini is the cosmic manifestation of divine energy at the base of the spinal column that is said to flow up certain subtle channels around the spine; the three psychic knots are the blocks we all have through our attachments to the material world; and *brahmi nadi* is the channel that carries the *kundalini* to her ultimate destination in the crown *chakra* on the top of the head.

STRENGTH AND STILLNESS THROUGH THE MIND

Meditation is a technique you can use to bring you much joy in life. It helps you to cultivate awareness, that is, your capacity to know, feel, and experience, and this enhanced awareness is vital for a vibrant, joyous, and fulfilled existence. As your awareness develops with practice you learn to sense more and more subtle physical and emotional tensions and you can respond to life with greater knowledge, strength, and sensitivity. You learn how to create strength and stillness through your mind.

We are the lucky recipients of the insights learned from millions of years of cumulative meditation practice by deeply spiritual souls. Many types of meditation have been taught that can lead us to the space of inner peace, whether through focusing on one part of the body, on the breath, on a symbol, on a mantra or word, or on a concept. The yogic tradition describes four consecutive and intertwined phases of meditation:

- ❀ **Sense withdrawal (*pratyahara*)** Removing your attention from external sense objects. This involves drawing your consciousness away from the material world as you internalize your awareness.
- ❀ **Concentration (*dharana*)** Holding one thought in your mind, but still being aware that you are meditating.
- ❀ **Meditation (*dhyana*)** More developed concentration, leading to an unbroken stream of consciousness.
- ❀ **Perfect equilibrium (*samadhi*)** Uniting of all forms of consciousness.

The difference between these states is that during the early phase of sense withdrawal you are still aware of and distracted by the outside world. All the sounds, feelings, images, tastes, and smells of life fill your body and head. Then, like a tortoise withdrawing its limbs, you leave your senses and enter the interior world of your consciousness.

In this vast internal cavern, you become aware of the contents of your mind: usually a random cacophony of past memories, impressions, and thoughts. To start the practice of concentration you need an object, say your breath, to focus on. In the early parts of this "internalizing" phase, you are conscious of meditating on your breath, and of yourself. The object of concentration (your breath), the meditator (you) and the act of meditation itself remain distinct. In this stage you can primarily focus on your breath, but you are also aware of your thoughts. It's a bit like watching a river of thoughts flow downstream.

As your concentration deepens it subtly evolves into a state of meditation where you become more absorbed in your breath. Your mind is filled only with the thoughts of your meditation and your breath, without interruption: how deep it is, how long it is, where you can feel it, and so on. You are now absorbed in a deeper form of concentration. When this stillness deepens further, the mind becomes single-focused and you effortlessly unite with the experienced object of your meditation, your breath. You are united with the universal consciousness, you are the breath, the breather, and the breathed—a literal integration known as *samadhi*, or perfect equilibrium.

You could say that this state of perfect equilibrium (*samadhi*) is perfected meditation (*dhyana*), meditation is improved concentration (*dharana*), and concentration grows out of internalizing your awareness (*pratyahara*) while focusing on one object. So, the meditative state is really perfected concentration; it is perfect awareness. But it's not always easy. As Arjuna, one of the greatest warriors of his time, said to Lord Krishna in the *Bhagavad Gita*, "The mind is restless, turbulent, and strong, as difficult to curb as the wind."

Your witnessing awareness

One of the main things you learn about in mediation is your "witnessing awareness." This is a very special part of your being that can literally watch your life, as if you are looking down from above at yourself. Connecting with your witnessing awareness also allows you to watch your habits and become aware of the inner essence of your being.

This is especially helpful because we all have patterns of thinking and behavior that lead to challenges in our lives. Some thought patterns can aggravae symptoms of illness, and some repeated behaviors can lead to repetitive complications. If you are skilled then you can get to know the pattern and "catch" it before it is enacted. If you are attentive you can learn how and when to choose the pattern and when to let it go. This path to skilful behavior is a continual journey that can be more or less painful depending on how aware you are and how deeply the pattern is engrained.

Living with your "witnessing awareness" allows you to be conscious of your present, to be aware of your inner patterns, and to watch your life. It gives you the gift of spontaneous clairvoyance, as though you can foresee your actions in any given moment. It removes the burden of knee-jerk compulsiveness and replaces it with an inner wisdom that can help you be aware of your feelings and thoughts, as well as the feelings and thoughts of others. This strength comes from clarity of awareness, which is best developed through the practice of Inner Silence (*see* Relationship, *Pukka Practice*, p.226).

MEDITATION TECHNIQUES
"Yoga is the cessation of the fluctuations of your mind."
PATANJALI'S YOGA SUTRAS

Just as we need to train our bodies to become strong, we need to train our mind to become still, and there are several techniques that we can use to help us.

Gazing (*trataka*)

This technique helps to develop your powers of concentration and visualization. When you have mastered this practice you can do creative visualizations, which are metaphorical journeys or imagined experiences that help you transform. This can be very useful for helping you "see" yourself behave in a certain way or do something that you want to achieve.

Place a candle on a small table, so that the flame is at eye level. Sit a few feet away and fix your concentration on the flame. It can be helpful to find the stillest point within the candle and focus on that. Try not to blink, and hold your concentrated gaze on the candle for about a minute. Your eyes might water a little. Close your eyes for a short while and hold the image of the flame in your "mind's eye." Repeat this process five times.

Eyebrow-center gazing (*shambhavi mudra*)

This is very useful for establishing you in the practice of watching the flow of your thoughts. Gazing in your eyebrow-center helps your mind to be single-focused.

Take a comfortable sitting position and turn your gaze to the tip of your nose. This will make you a little cross-eyed. Hold the focus for a few seconds. Raise the eyes slightly, so that this cross-eyed gaze now falls directly between the eyebrows. After a few more seconds, close your eyes and hold this focus on your eyebrow-center internally. Hold this concentration for several minutes.

Meditation on the breath (*prana vidya*)

This is at the heart of many meditation techniques. Its simplicity is its beauty, its omnipresence its subtlety. This practice has so many layers of ever-illuminating depth that it can be practiced forever. As well as taking you on a journey to a place of inner stillness, it has the wonderful side effect of being deeply relaxing.

Sit comfortably. Feel yourself in your seat. Put down roots below, become steady above. Do a brief "body-scan" and soften any tension: feet-legs-hips-back-spine-shoulders-neck-back of head-top of head-forehead-eyelids-ears-nose-mouth-whole face-throat-chest-belly. Notice your breath and let it flow in and out. Let any immediate thoughts flow away. Feel your stability and strength. Feel how much you are caring for yourself.

Choose a place in your body—perhaps the tip of the nose, in the chest, or in the belly—to watch your breath and use the same place in every practice. (Consistency is vital for making progress in your technique.) Feel your breath flowing in with each inhalation and flowing out with each exhalation. Feel it touch your skin, feel it expand your whole body. Let your breath expand. Feel it swelling. Feel it moving. Now watch it leave, feel it soften. In and out; in and out. Notice how deeply you are breathing, notice how quickly you are breathing.

As you journey into the practice, watch your breath change, deepen, slow; observe the ebb and flow of your breath, rising and falling, expanding and contracting. Feel the pulse of your breath, sound the pulse of your life. Let any wandering thoughts flow away. Watch them and let them go with no judgment. Come back to your breath. It's an eternal practice: no forcing, no effort—just watching. Do whatever feels good for you right now. There is no right or wrong. When your mind wanders just bring it back to the stream of your breath at the center of your attention. Breathe.

*"Let go of your worries
and be completely clear-hearted,
like the face of a mirror
that contains no images.
If you want a clear mirror,
behold yourself
and see the shameless truth,
which the mirror reflects.
If metal can be polished
to a mirror-like finish,
what polishing might the mirror
of the heart require?
Between the mirror and the heart
is this single difference:
the heart conceals secrets,
while the mirror does not."*

**MAWLANA JALAL-AL-DIN RUMI,
THIRTEENTH-CENTURY POET
AND SUFI MYSTIC**

THE BEST RELAXING HERBS

There is a vast range of herbs that have a longstanding use for nourishing the nervous system and helping us relax. Those that I use regularly in my clinic include oatstraw flowering tops, skullcap, passion flower, lavender, and rose, but those listed below are my favorites. *See* The Pukka Pantry for full details.

Ashwagandha (*Withania somnifera*) This herb has incredible nourishing abilities that help our body cope with stress and is used whenever there is any sign of deficiency, coldness, or weakness leading to tiredness or debility. This makes ashwagandha the herb of choice when there is any chronic imbalance that results in depletion and convalescence. Its grounding and stabilizing effects help in treating insomnia, palpitations, and anxiety.

Brahmi (*Bacopa monnieri*) The cooling properties of this herb are useful for addressing signs of mental or emotional imbalance. I specifically think of using brahmi whenever there is nervous depletion resulting from mental attachment to a redundant and nonhealth-inducing pattern of behavior, such as addiction to alcohol, foods, or unhelpful emotional habits.

Chamomile (*Matricaria recutita*) This herb is also known as German Chamomile (and not to be confused with Roman Chamomile [*Anthemis nobilis*], which is really very bitter). It is virtually impossible to talk about relaxing herbs without mentioning chamomile. It is traditionally used for fair-skinned people who are prone to anxiety and are emotionally vulnerable. Chamomile is especially delicious as a tea.

Gotu kola (*Hydrocotyle asiatica*) This herb is true food for the mind. Its greatest asset is its ability to penetrate deeply into the circulatory system and carry its consciousness-enhancing properties into the brain. Gotu kola relaxes the channels of circulation, allowing more blood to flow, whether this is needed for nutrition or for wound healing. It is particularly useful when relaxation is needed in order to think more clearly.

Tulsi (*Ocimum sanctum*) Also known as Holy Basil, tulsi has recently become one of my favorite herbs for relaxing the nervous system. Although it is also good for immunity, its light aromatic scent is wonderful for lifting the spirits, and alleviating depression. It is packed with essential oils that help to open the lungs, remove grief, and relax tension. It is also very useful for relieving insomnia and tension headaches.

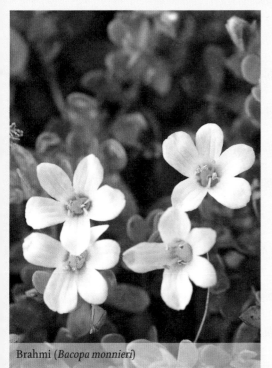

Brahmi (*Bacopa monnieri*)

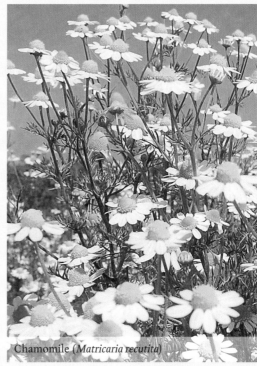

Chamomile (*Matricaria recutita*)

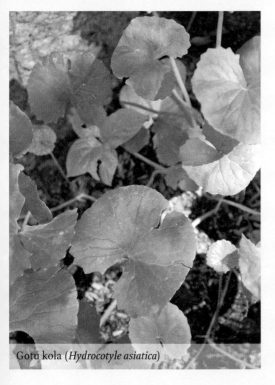

Gotu kola (*Hydrocotyle asiatica*)

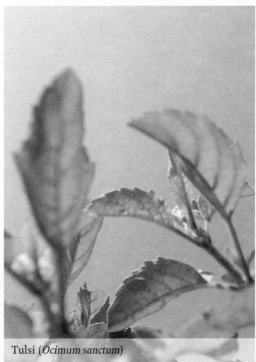

Tulsi (*Ocimum sanctum*)

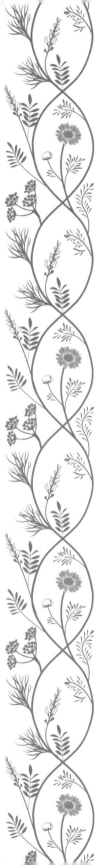

PUKKA PRACTICE

A SELF-MASSAGE ROUTINE AND YOGA NIDRA

The healing power of touch should never be underestimated. This delicious practice loosens toxins, clears tensions, and rejuvenates your whole body and mind. The most beneficial oil is sesame oil that has been briefly heated to boiling temperature, called "cured sesame oil," which increases its antioxidant and healing properties. Olive oil and coconut oil are also very nourishing.

Yoga Nidra is a deep relaxation practice devised by Swami Satyananda Saraswati, the great Indian saint and yoga teacher. Your body rests while your mind remains awake, which allows you to relax on a deep, cellular level. Yoga Nidra takes you on a journey through your senses, body, breath, mind, and heart—the fundamental elements of life – to the very essence of your inner being. You can either get a friend to read this to you, or you can record it and play it back to yourself. Better still, you can buy a fuller version of Yoga Nidra on CD (*see* Resources, p.251).

Body massage

First warm the oil by placing the bottle in an airing cupboard or in a pan of hot water. Sit or stand on an old towel in a warm room, out of any drafts.

Massage the oil into your entire body, beginning at the feet and working up the legs toward the middle of the body and then up your arms. Work the oil deeply into your skin. Use long strokes on the limbs and circular strokes on the joints. Massage the abdomen and chest in broad, clockwise, circular motions; on the abdomen, follow the path of the large intestine, moving up on the right side, then across beneath your ribs, then down on the left side. Also massage the oil into your scalp, back of your neck, and into your ears (but not if you have an ear infection). Apply some warm oil to the crown of your head in circular strokes. Massage with care and patience for 5 to 20 minutes; then allow the skin to digest the oil.

After the oil has been absorbed deeply (20 to 30 minutes), have a warm bath or shower. (Take care as the oil on your feet can make it easy to slip.) There is no need to use soap but you may want to wash your hair. Dry yourself with a clean towel.

Apply a constitutionally appropriate organic essential oil to your wrists, neck, throat, and "third eye" (in between your eyebrows): patchouli, chamomile, or lavender for *vata*; ylang ylang, neroli, or rose otto for *pitta*; frankincense, cardamom, or cinnamon for *kapha*. Make sure you stay warm after your massage.

Yoga Nidra

Lie on your back with your arms by your side. Start to become aware of the parts of your body that are touching the ground beneath you. Imagine that you are lying on a dry, soft, green bed of moss. This moss is holding your body, absorbing your contours, allowing you to rest comfortably. Now take your awareness to your breath: allow each exhalation to flow long and deeply and let go of any anxiety or tiredness. Feel your body sinking more heavily into the floor.

Turn to the senses. Starting with hearing, become aware of any natural or mechanical sounds; let them come, until you are aware of the subtle sound of your own breath. Stay with the hearing for a few moments. Next, turn your awareness to touch. Become aware of the parts of the body that are touching each other: the toes, fingers, lips, eyelids. Feel your clothes touching your body. Now move to an awareness of sight. Notice the kaleidoscopic images appearing on the back of your eyelids, a plethora of colors and patterns arising from your memory. Then become aware of taste. Notice the quality in your mouth: moisture, taste, temperature, and if there are any flavors. (You may need to swallow for this.) Finally, bring your awareness to the sense of smell. Notice any particular aromas in the air. Fine-tune your awareness of smell as you breathe up and down the length of the body. As you inhale feel this pressure ascend and, as you exhale, feel it descend, at the same time experiencing a "letting go," a release on the exhalation.

Making your resolve

The next part of the practice is the formation of your *sankalpa*, an intention or a resolve. It is a BIG intention, your life-long goal. This *sankalpa* is the seed for how you would like your life to develop. As you say your *sankalpa* silently to yourself you can imagine walking in a newly ploughed field and, as you repeat it, see yourself planting this seed into fresh, fertile soil. Repeat your *sankalpa* three times.

The next stage is to circulate your awareness around the different areas of the body in a "body-scan," silently naming each individual body part, taking your awareness there and trying to visualize that part. Despite the deep relaxation that this induces you must remain awake throughout. Start with the right side of the body: silently name the thumb, each finger, the palm and back of the hand, wrist, elbow, shoulder, and so on until you reach your feet. Go slowly. Next, move your awareness to the left-hand side of your body, following the same "body-scan." Now move your awareness to the back of the body, and name, become aware of and visualize each body part. Feel the length of the whole spine, moving your awareness up and down, and then up to the top of your head. Become aware of the hair on your head, the forehead, the right and left temples, right and left cheeks, and so on until you have named every part of the head. Now move down the front

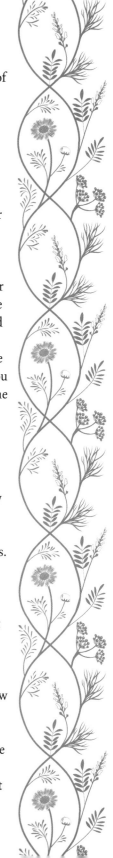

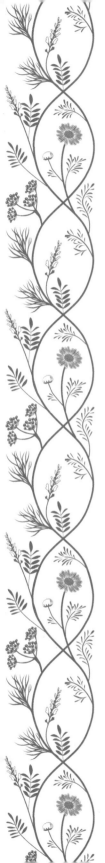

of the torso: collarbones, chest, diaphragm, lower abdomen. Lastly, move your awareness inside your body, to your heart, lungs, liver, your digestive system, reproductive system, and your brain. Move your awareness to the outside of your body again and integrate all of these separate individual parts by repeating silently to yourself, "the whole body, the whole body, the whole body …"

Remaining awake, start to experience different sensations: density, temperature, and emotion. Feel the sensation of heaviness in your body, as though you are made of solid rock, that you are fixed to the earth. Now leave that sensation and exchange it for its opposite, lightness. Feel that your whole body is filled with millions of tiny air molecules that are floating up to the surface of your body. Next, move on to another sensation: temperature. Imagine that you are outside on a cold winter's day. Visualize the color blue and feel that each breath you take in is cold. Now swap this sensation for its opposite, heat. You are outside on a warm summer's day; the sun's rays are warming your whole body. Visualize the color red and feel that the air you breath in is heating your body. Now bring your focus to your emotions. Recall a moment in your life when you felt sad and, acting as a distant observer, recall this moment of sadness. What does it feel like? Where do you feel it? What quality does this feeling of sadness have? Leave this sensation and exchange it for its opposite, happiness, and ask yourself the same questions.

Leave this memory of happiness and keep your attention on your breath. Inhale from the tip of your nostrils up to the eyebrow center and into the center of your brain and breath out from the center of your brain to the tip of your nostrils. Follow this pathway for five complete breaths. As an extension of this exercise, move your awareness to the tips of your toes. Start an imaginary practice so that when you inhale, you breath in from the tips of your toes and the breath travels up the front plane of your body until the breath reaches the top of your head. When you exhale, breathe along the back plane of the body and out through the heels. As you breathe in, draw in anything positive in the universe that you need in your life; as you exhale, let go of and breathe away anything that you do not need in your life. Start to see the flow of the breath as a stream of golden light.

Your visualization

Leave this awareness and, remaining awake, bring your attention to the space behind the eyebrow-center, the *chidakasha*, the space of consciousness. Start to become aware of the infinite space expanding there. Now begin a visualization. See yourself setting out on a walk one day. As you are walking along the lush green path, you are aware of the soft ground beneath you, the valley around you, and the freshness in the air. After a little way you come to a field. You bend down and pick up some soil and you smell the fertile, nutritious earth. You know that you are made up from the elements of the earth—it gives you structure, solidity, and strength. You put down the earth and continue your walk. You see a small stream that is trickling by and you hear its sound, smell its freshness, feel the cool water cleansing your face. As you drink some you feel it refresh and cleanse you inside. You know this water exists in your body—it gives you moisture and fluidity and "glues" you together. Carry on, passing by trees and fields and hearing birdsong.

After a while you come to a small fire. You feel its warmth filling your body, see the light spreading in every direction. As you sit by the fire you fall into a deep meditation in which you feel calm, serene, and full of peace. You know that this fire exists in your body, bringing you warmth, light, and energy. Then you slowly carry on your journey and after a little while you enter a disused railroad tunnel. You can see the end where it is light. You can feel a wind blowing into the tunnel and become aware of its qualities: light, erratic, cold, drying. You know that this wind moves in your body—it is a messenger, a carrier, the force of movement. You carry on walking and at the end of the tunnel you become aware that you have entered an open valley. It is a huge space. You can see for miles and you become aware of the qualities of space, its pervasiveness and openness—it is the arena in which you live. You become aware of all the space in your body: your hollow organs, the space inbetween your joints. You feel at peace in this mighty expanse.

Now return to an awareness of the *chidakasha*, the quiet, dark place behind the eyebrow-center. You exist in this calm space, feeling at ease and peaceful. Feel the deep peace emanating from you. Deep, deep peace. Picture yourself watering the seeds you planted at the beginning of this practice and repeat your *sankalpa* three times, feeling that the intentions of your heart will bear fruit.

As you near the end of the practice, slowly start to externalize your awareness by noticing the different sounds that you can hear: your own breath, sounds inside this room, and outside it. Then become aware of different sensations: your clothes touching your skin, the temperature of the air surrounding you, the stillness in your body. Come to focus on the back of the eyelids and become aware of colors, patterns, shapes. Next come down to your mouth again and swallow to become aware of the flavors in your mouth and then, moving to your nose, become aware of any particular smells. Now take a couple of deep breaths, breathing up and down the body, slowly externalizing your awareness. Recall the bed of green moss that you were lying on. Remember where you are; feel grounded and stable. Start to make some delicate movements, slowly waking your body up. Now have a stretch in any direction you want, waking your body up, feeling refreshed and awake. Come back to your space.

Hari om tat sat ("Universal consciousness is infinite spirit—that is the truth").

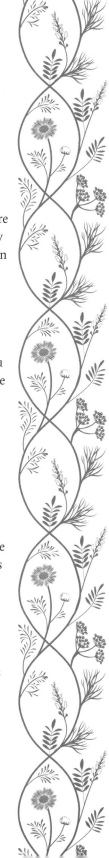

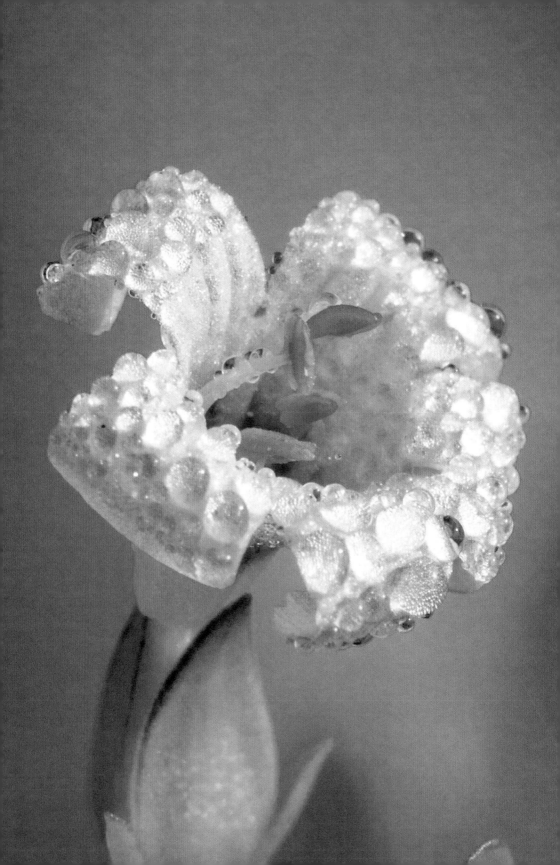

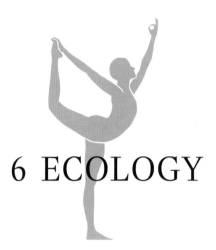

6 ECOLOGY

"The essence of all beings is Earth. The essence of the Earth is Water. The essence of Water is plants. The essence of plants is the human being ..."
CHANDOGYA UPANISHAD

We can't talk about our own health without understanding our place in our environment, because in order to fulfill our potential we have to live in the context of our surroundings. We have to know our place in the ecosystem of which we are a part, and this means living "consciously": being aware of nature and how it affects us and how we, in turn, affect nature. We need to ask what we require from the world around us so that we can flourish—but we also need to identify what we can give back. We are all interconnected, and Ayurveda helps us weave this ecological web.

THE ECOLOGY OF HEALTH

Our well-being and the health of our ecosystem are intimately linked: both relate to the sustainability of our lives. To be truly sustainable, we have to be aware of the needs of our environment. This requires deep ecological awareness, which in essence is deep spiritual awareness. By looking at how Ayurveda understands nature, the life force, and the disease process and how we can connect with nature through living as sustainably as possible, we can create a profound spiritual awareness of the ecology of our health.

Just as we are a part of the ecosystem, it is a part of us, and this unity reflects the interconnected nature of consciousness. Metaphorically, nature is the field in which we can experience consciousness. We need to nurture, tend, and replant this field if we are to be nourished enough to experience a spiritual dimension to our lives. This nurturing is dependent upon the choices we make in how we live. It comes down to how aware we are of our place in the ecosystem and how conscious we are of what it is that infuses us with life.

Another way of looking at our place in nature is through the concept of "holons," as discussed by the philosopher Ken Wilber. Holons are evolving systems where everything is growing together as an integrated whole. This theory describes nature in terms of its duality: every organism or idea is both a whole in its own right as well as a part of another whole. You can visualize this in terms of Russian dolls, where each complete doll is contained within another. The concept can also be understood by thinking of written language, where a letter is itself a letter, as well as a part of a word that forms part of a sentence, that makes up a paragraph, that creates a chapter, that becomes a book, which is part of the whole form of literature within that language.

These analogies of interconnection continue throughout the natural world: a seed makes a seedling, which grows into a shrub, which grows into a tree, which is part of a forest that forms part of the ecosystem. It is the same with the human world: the individual is a part of a family, that is part of a community, that is part of a society, that is within a culture, that is within all the cultures of the world. We have to know the characteristics and needs of each component to understand the whole. It's no good only understanding ourselves divorced from the values of our family and culture. This will create friction.

These ever-expanding circles of inclusion continue within Ayurveda: your individual constitution (*dosha*) is formed from the five natural elements (*see* the next page), which are contained within your mind, which is contained within the energy of nature, which evolves from universal consciousness.

I find this thought process invaluable in helping to create an inclusive attitude to life. Every part of us is essential to our total wholeness, warts and all. If we look at something in isolation we are missing our perspective of the whole. We are not integrating our total being.

The material world

To understand fully how Ayurveda relates to you, it is essential to grasp its view of our ecosystem. It considers that the world we live in—the material world—is made from "building blocks" that evolve through increasing concentrations of density, from subtle energy to gross matter. These building blocks are known as the "Five Great Elements," the primordial constituents of the world: Ether, Air, Fire, Water and Earth. These express the natural qualities of spaciousness, movement, heat, fluidity, and solidity, which allow us to hear, touch, see, taste, and smell. Every idea in Ayurveda is based on these fundamental elements, and you will find out more about them as you read on.

The five elements combine in different proportions to make up the physical universe, which includes the natural world, our body, and our mind. They are the materials that make up the three constitutional *doshas* (*vata, pitta,* and *kapha*), as well as the qualities of nature that determine the taste and energetic properties of herbs and foods: ginger is hot because of the fire element; cucumbers are juicy because of the water element, and so on. If you can learn to observe, understand, and develop a language for these elements, then you can describe the energy and quality of anything in nature. You will have the vocabulary to interpret the holons of your life.

THE FIVE GREAT ELEMENTS

The essence of each of the Five Great Elements (known in Sanskrit as *panchamahabhuta*) can be more fully understood by looking in detail at what they are and what they represent. Try and see their qualities in yourself, your friends, and the world around you. It is important to note that the Ayurvedic elements do not equate to the periodic elements of modern chemistry; the elements are more closely associated with "states" of matter.

Ether (*akasa*): the principle of all-pervasive potential

Natural qualities Expansive, light, subtle, clear, cold, infinite, and all-encompassing space. *Vata* is an expression of Ether.
Sense Sound
Organ Ear

According to Ayurveda's "Big Bang" theory, Ether (also called Space) grows out of universal consciousness and develops into the subtle quality of awareness. Ether is the arena within which life takes place and it holds all the potential for life to manifest and be experienced. It is this emptiness of space that gives us the potential to empower our lives by using our awareness to make choices. Unfortunately, we are often duped by our senses into believing that the world is "solid" and "full" and that there is reduced space for us to fulfil our potential.

The Five Great Elements and the *dosha*s
Vata Ether and Air
Pitta Fire and Water
Kapha Water and Earth

Space is everywhere: in our minds, lungs, intestines, bladder, in between cells, within cells, within atoms. Consider the atomic particles that make up objects. They are in perpetual motion; it is just their density that creates the illusion of solidity. Even this book, supposedly solid, is made from persistently moving particles. Our potential lies in realizing the possibilities available within this space and within us.

The qualities of *vata* are an expression of Ether; it is why *vata* is light, sensitive, cold, creative, and can be "spaced out."

Ether allows the subtle element of sound to emerge out of its inherent silence and to travel through it: there is no sound without space. The vibrational frequencies of sounds differ and not all of them can be heard by everyone. Humans, dolphins, dogs, and bats all have different sensitivities to the various pitches emerging out of the great universal orchestra. What can be heard by one cannot be heard by another. The expression of Ether reminds us that reality is entirely in the mind of the perceiver. It is unique and individual.

✳ Air (*vayu*): the principle of motion
Natural qualities Like the wind, light, mobile, clear, rough, dry, and erratic. *Vata* is an expression of Air.
Sense Touch
Organ Skin

Ether contains the element of Air, creating the potential for movement and change. The perpetual state of motion and adaptation is due to Air, as it takes on a material form that rolls from one state into another: embryo to baby to child to adult. It is always moving: electrons whizz around nuclei, chemical messages move between cells, blood pumps through our veins, breath moves through the lungs, our thoughts perpetually chatter. Outside, the rotation of the Earth creates night and day, equinoxes, eclipses, and seasonal changes. The obvious connection between the Air—the principle of movement—and the gaseous exchange that occurs as part of cellular respiration represents the vital, life-giving importance of this element.

As well as being an expression of Ether, *vata* also reflects the qualities of Air. It is why *vata* is always on the move, can be erratic, and develops dry and rough skin.

The element of Air enables us to experience the feeling of touch. Sensations of temperature, pressure, or humidity travel through the receptors in the skin via the nervous system to the brain. Every signal in the universe, be it sound, touch, light, warmth, taste, or smell, is carried by the Air element.

✳ Fire (*tejas*): the principle of illumination
Natural qualities Hot, sharp, fluid, penetrating, luminous, light, ascending, and dispersing. *Pitta* is an expression of Fire.
Sense Sight
Organ Eyes

Air creates the element of Fire, as it combusts out of the friction created by movement through the Ether. And having been born, fire burns brightly: the fierce progress of a meteor ablaze through our atmosphere creates fire and light.

Fire converts solid matter to liquids and then to gas, and also transforms cold to hot: fire burns wood, which melts ice into water, which heats up and eventually evaporates. There is no greater example of the Fire element than our sun: a giant furnace large enough to hold a million Earths and burning at 25 million°F at its core, it lights our day and creates life.

"Fire" is present in our digestive systems in the form of the enzymes that transform food into fuel for our tissues, organs, and cells. This is why Ayurveda uses the term "digestive fire" (*agni*) as an analogy for our digestive health. The energy-production centers in the body are the mitochondria in our cells, which manifest the quality of Fire as they combust nutritional potential to create cellular energy. The Fire element transforms potential energy to kinetic energy, giving off heat and light in the process, which keeps our bodies at a constant 98.6°F.

Pitta is an expression of Fire, as it has the tendency to be hot, sharp, intelligent and passionate.

Fire is connected to the subtle element of sight. It allows us to perceive the light of the universe through our eyes due to the metabolic activity of light-sensitive photons in the retina. Again, different animals can perceive different frequencies of light, so visual experience is not the same: bees see in hexagons, dogs see mainly in black and white, and some birds see in a range of colors broader than our rainbow. The world is truly just as you perceive it.

Water (*jala*): the principle of cohesion

Natural qualities Fluid, heavy, wet, lubricating, cool, soft, cohesive, and stable. *Pitta* and *kapha* are expressions of Water.
Sense Taste
Organ Tongue

Water is created when Fire liquefies certain substances; it is a by-product as they cool and condense. Water is the "glue" of life that holds everything together; cement and sand are of no use without it. It has the ability to bind and attract, as water's fluid cohesiveness brings everything it touches into one whole. In this sense it is responsible for the quality of friendship and love. It creates a continuum: water, rain, river, sea. The Earth's surface is predominantly water, and both plants and humans consist of about 60 percent water. Water is essential for life, as it lubricates our mucous membranes, fills the cells, and creates a continuous sequence throughout the entire body.

The Water element is expressed in the fluid and oily nature of *pitta*'s potential for greasy skin, as well as in the liquid nature of wet, cool, and heavy *kapha*.

Water relates to the subtle element of taste. It allows us to experience the flavor of the world: flavors are only detectable when the tongue is wet. Salt encourages the secretion of saliva, which is why it makes food tastier.

✤ Earth (*prithvi*): the principle of stability

Natural qualities Thick, dense, solid, hard, heavy, and stable. *Kapha* is an expression of Earth.
Sense Smell
Organ Nose

In Ayurvedic thinking, the material world is merely a condensation of consciousness. The Water element creates the possibility for consciousness to become denser, giving the appearance of "solidity" as it condenses into the element of Earth. The Earth element gives structure to matter, so that there are defined objects with boundaries, form, and shape. Muscles and bones are high in the Earth element, as they give us strength and structure. Of course, this illusion of solidity is not absolute, because the nature of the universe is empty and within every object is Ether (Space)—even the chair you are sitting on.

Kapha is an expression of the Earth element through the thick, hard, and dense qualities that give the *dosha* such solidity.

The subtle element of Earth is the sense of smell. Earthy and dense objects emit aromas that are carried to us by the wind. What better smell is there than the earth after rain? Smell is the essence of the Earth element, helping us to be reminded of the past and feel grounded in the present: hot toast, fresh roses, lavender ...

Ether

Earth

Air

Water Fire

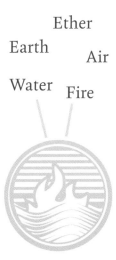

NATURAL QUALITIES OF THE ELEMENTS

Quality	Element(s)	Action	Effect on *dosha*	Example
Heat	Fire	Heating, digestive, moves upward and outward, diaphoretic (causes excess sweating)	Increases *pitta*; reduces *vata* and *kapha*	Ginger, garlic, chile, pippali, alcohol
Lightness	Fire, Air, Ether	Easy to digest, reduces accumulations and weight	Increases *vata*; reduces *pitta* and *kapha*	Popcorn, rice, black pepper, gotu kola
Dryness	Earth, Air	Drying, astringent, dehydrating, causes constipation	Increases *vata* and *kapha*; reduces *pitta*	Millet, guggul, strong tea, coffee
Penetrating/ sharp	Fire	Enters deeply into the body and mind, with immediate effect	Increases *vata* and *pitta*; reduces *kapha*	Alcohol, cannabis, salt, vacha
Smooth	Water	Eases tension, brings together, reduces roughness	Increases *pitta* and *kapha*; reduces *vata*	Sesame oil, ghee
Stable	Earth	Encourages relaxation, can create sluggishness in excess	Increases *kapha*; reduces *vata* and *pitta*	Yogurt, candies, ashwagandha
Soft	Water	Eases tension, increases tenderness, reduces hardness, pacifies	Increases *pitta* and *kapha*; reduces *vata*	Oats, ghee, avocado, marshmallow root, licorice
Liquid/fluid	Water	Holds together, lubricates and moistens	Increases *pitta* and *kapha;* reduces *vata*	Water, fruit and vegetable juices, aloe vera juice
Subtle	Air	Penetrates deeply into the tissues, expansive, increases awareness	Increases *vata* and *pitta*; reduces *kapha*	Brahmi, ghee, honey, alcohol
Slimy	Water	Heals broken bones, soothes, plasters skin, creates lack of clarity in excess	Increases *pitta* and *kapha;* reduces *vata*	Oil, oats, shatavari

Quality	Element(s)	Action	Effect on *dosha*	Example
Cold	Water	Cooling, slows digestion, contracting, moves inward and downward, restrains	Increases *vata* and *kapha*; reduces *pitta*	Neem, mint, wheat
Heavy	Earth, Water	Difficult to digest, builds tissues, moves down, nourishes, in excess creates tiredness	Increases *kapha*; reduces *vata* and *pitta*	Yogurt, meat, ashwagandha
Greasy/ unctuous	Water	Difficult to digest, lubricating, nourishing, increases love, moistening	Increases *pitta* and *kapha*; reduces *vata*	Oils, nuts, shatavari
Dull/ sluggish	Earth, Water	Increases tissues, causes stagnation, slowness, pacifies	Increases *kapha*; reduces *vata* and *pitta*	Tofu, yogurt, nutmeg
Rough	Air	Reduces lubrication, causes dry skin, brittle bones, increases inflexibility, scrapes	Increases *vata*; reduces *pitta* and *kapha*	Popcorn, triphala
Mobile	Air	Encourages movement and changeability, releases	Increases *vata* and *pitta*; reduces *kapha*	Spices, chile
Hard	Earth	Difficult to digest, gives strength	Increases *vata* and *kapha*; reduces *pitta*	Nuts, coconut, almonds, sesame seeds
Solid/ dense	Earth	Difficult to digest, increases structural strength, mental fortitude	Increases *kapha*; reduces *vata* and *pitta*	Root vegetables, cheese
Gross	Earth	Difficult to digest, causes obstructions	Increases *kapha*; reduces *vata* and *pitta*	Ashwagandha, meat, mushrooms
Clear	Air, Space	Increases clarity	Increases *vata* and *pitta*; reduces *kapha*	Sprouted beans, brahmi

THE LIFE FORCE (*PRANA*) AND THE ECOSYSTEM

"The broadest meaning of the word prana *is 'force of energy'. In this sense, the universe is filled with* prana; *all creation is a manifestation of force, a play of force. Everything that was, is, or shall be, is nothing but the different modes of expression of the universal force."*
PARAMAHAMSA YOGANANDA, YOGI AND SAINT

The central path to understanding the ecosystem is the experience of the life force, the vitalistic principle of nature that animates the world and brings the elements to life. One of the most wonderful and profound teachings of Ayurveda—in fact, of all traditional medical systems—is the notion of a life force that pervades all existence. As mentioned earlier, in Ayurveda it is known as *prana*.

Everything that is alive is energized by *prana*. The fresh vitality after a summer rainstorm, the energy of a waterfall, the tingling in the hands after a clear meditation, the deep nourishment of a fresh meal, the sweet vitality of feeling love—these are all living experiences of the life force. Within you, *prana* brings immunity, warmth, strength, enthusiasm, and glow, protecting you from infections, holding muscles in place, and bringing a sparkle to your eyes and peace to your heart. *Prana* enables balance, rhythm, and homeostasis, giving you the ability to regulate your life, from your in-breath to your out-breath, to the harmonious rhythm of your heartbeat, to eating food, and passing wastes. In essence, it brings vitality, enthusiasm, and life itself. This life force empowers your entire ecology, as it permeates every molecule of matter.

The life force is like a current of electricity, which is demonstrated clearly in the lifecycle of plants. Green plants, trees, grasses, herbs, and vegetables all harvest the sun's life force as light via the process of photosynthesis. When we consume these foods, this stored solar energy is released into our bodies as electrons. It is then transformed into the biological energy necessary for all cellular function: we can live. This is the journey of the life force from the sun, through nature, into our bodies. As the Nobel Prize-winning biochemist Albert Szent-Györgyi said, "We live by a small trickle of electricity from the sun."

Above and beyond the miracle of germination, growth, maturity, fruiting, and spreading seeds, plants are the basis of human life, health, and wealth. Plants bring us clothes, food, building, and warmth. It is their *prana*, their vibrant vitality, that allows us to live, rivers to be purified, and land to be remineralized. This is the power of the life force: it enables us to live and experience our part in the whole.

There are three ways to get more *prana* into your life: through food, through *qigong* or yoga exercises, and through breathing practices. And nothing has more *prana* than green foods (*see* box below), especially "superfoods," such as wheatgrass juice, sprouted seeds, spirulina, and chlorella (*see* p.190). They have trapped higher-than-average amounts of solar energy, which is released into our body after eating, their photovoltaic electrons freed to recharge our overworked bodies and rejuvenate our minds. As is written in the sixteenth-century Indian text, *Vrikshayurveda*, "Knowing this truth, one should undertake planting of trees, since trees yield the means of attaining the four goals of life: *dharma* (life purpose), *artha* (wealth), *kama* (pleasure) and *moksa* (enlightenment)."

Chlorophyll: nature's life force food

The "green" in green plants comes from chlorophyll and brings a wealth of revitalizing properties. Specifically chlorophyll:

Rejuvenates Chlorophyll helps to renew tissues and organs. Its high levels of RNA and DNA nucleic acids nourish cellular renewal, thus helping to delay aging. Chlorophyll's ability to neutralize oxidative stressors means that it can reduce chemical and environmental oxidative damage and help to increase vitality. By normalizing intestinal flora, it assists digestion and improves absorption.

Alkalizes Green foods help the blood remain at the healthy pH of 7.2. Our acidic diet (from meat, dairy, sugar, alcohol, and grains) means the body has to compensate by leaching vital minerals and other nutrients to achieve this alkaline state.

Mineralizes Chlorophyll is made in plants that are also high in trace minerals such as magnesium (essential for relaxing muscles and reducing blood pressure and food cravings) and zinc (essential for the bones, nerves, and immunity).

Builds blood There are many reasons why green plants can be considered "blood-building" foods, but perhaps the most interesting is the similarity in the structures of their respective colored pigments, chlorophyll (in plants) and hem (in blood). The biological relationship between these two molecules remains unclear, but it appears that small amounts of the digestive products of chlorophyll stimulate the synthesis of either hem or globin (or both) in animals and humans, resulting in more hemoglobin.

Detoxifies Chlorophyll positively affect all the organs of detoxification (the bowels, liver, mucous membranes, and blood cells). It also has the ability to neutralize toxic cellular agents, including free radicals, environmental pollutants, and carcinogens.

Purifies the intestines Parsley is renowned for sweetening the breath, and other chlorophyll-rich foods clear bacterial overgrowth and reduce yeasts and other fungi in your digestive system. Chlorophyll prevents putrification throughout the body, clearing noxious smells from your "hollow" organs: the stomach, intestines, bowels, and lungs.

Reduces inflammation Green foods specifically reduce inflammation throughout the digestive tract, liver, pancreas, and joints. Chlorophyll strongly opposes the heat and inflammation associated with radiation and chemotherapy.

HERBAL SUSTAINABILITY

It is remarkable, but perhaps not surprising, to think that most herbs are harvested from the wild. Have you ever thought where your last cup of elderflower, licorice or lime flowers came from? These herbs are rarely cultivated, as they are so readily available for free in the local environment. This means that herb collectors go out into the forests to pick what they need. Herb collectors in the countries where many Ayurvedic herbs are grown are usually the poorest of the poor. They often do not own land and are dependent on annual wild herb harvests to supplement their income. However, unregulated harvesting is putting the sustainability of herbs—and, by extension, herbal medicines—into question.

In January 2004, Alan Hamilton, a plant specialist working with the World Wildlife Fund, released a paper on the threat to the herbal community from the indiscriminate overharvesting of medicinal herbs. He noted that approximately 75 percent of all medicinal herbs come from the wild; there are 50,000 species that are used as medicines and 10,000 of these are threatened. This means that a staggering twenty percent of all herbal species used throughout the world are under threat! When so many species are harvested without regulation and in such large volumes, this puts natural plant populations under increasing pressure. For example, *Echinacea angustifolia*, goldenseal, devil's claw, guggul, sandalwood, American ginseng, and slippery elm are all currently threatened in their natural habitats.

Wild herbs

The reliance of herbal medicine on wild herbs is due to the fact that many plants often require very specific habitats, making them difficult to cultivate. Herb prices worldwide are also very low, which means there is little incentive for farmers to grow herbs rather than conventional food crops. Some herbal authorities also consider herbs grown in the wild to be more potent, reflected in their higher price: the cost of wild American ginseng is 30 percent higher than that of the cultivated plant. This makes sense if you consider that the healing properties of plants are often related to their own ability to protect themselves from the sorts of invading bacteria and fungi that are rife in the wild. Because organic farming replicates a "wild" environment to a certain degree, it is also why organic food is better for you.

The threat to herbal supplies

It is estimated that the Ayurvedic pharmacopoeia includes upwards of 1,250 species, with approximately 300 of these in regular demand. Similar figures exist for Chinese, North American, and Western herbal medicine. In India and Sri Lanka most herbs come from the wild: in excess of 90 percent of herbal material used in Ayurveda comes from the forests, mountains, and plains of the Indian subcontinent and is sourced in an unregulated manner. In other parts of the world there is similar pressure, with 80 percent of species coming from the wild in China and up to 99 percent in Africa. Global demand for herbal medicine has increased by an estimated ten to twenty percent per annum in the last decade and so the pressures to overharvest are immense.

However, the harvesting of wild herbs is a relatively accessible source of income for people without land or a regular job. Herbs grow for free in the wild and trading collected wild plants can support a family. In the higher-altitude region of Nepal all families harvest herbs and it can account for 15–30 percent of their income.

The escalating demand for herbal medicine coupled with the needs of low-income families puts increasing pressure on natural habitats. Having been involved in trying to grow jatamansi and kutki in the Himalaya, I have seen these pressures first hand, as the local pickers trot down the hillsides laden with unsustainably harvested wild herbs. Instead of waiting until the right time to start wild collection, they have now become involved in a race to get to the herbs before other collectors. It is common to see people harvesting some species three months before the traditional time, at the very period when the plants can form seeds and thereby guarantee their future. The precious jewels of the land are being stripped.

The organic solution

So what is the future for herbal medicine and Ayurveda? As discussed earlier, organic foods and herbs have higher levels of secondary metabolite compounds than conventionally grown crops (*see* Nourishment, p.62). It is these secondary metabolites that give the plants their therapeutic taste and phytonutrients, which means the energetic qualities of organic plants are potentially more potent and thus more effective.

Organic certification also necessitates a deeper relationship between the farmer and the buyer. Because of the legal requirements, including testing for contaminants (toxic elements and pesticide residues), it is necessary to have very close contact with the source of the plants to ensure quality, consistency, and documentation. The transparency of the farming practices allows consumers to see how each species is handled, what inputs have been added, and that appropriate checks on quality have taken place. At Pukka Herbs, we have established detailed practices and an organic certification system that brings benefits to the farmer, plant quality, and the end user. Through this system we know the name of the farmer, the exact location of cultivation, and the date of harvest for all the organically certified species that we produce. This evolving process has led to a much deeper confidence that nature is respected, that the farmers are well treated and that the Ayurvedic plants we produce are of the highest quality.

The future

The majority of herbal species are not on the verge of extinction but many are threatened. We, as supporters of the herbal community and, therefore, bearers of their heritage, must make sure that we act in a truly Ayurvedic fashion and help to prevent "disease" before there is a problem. We should therefore use herbs, oils, and foods that aim to conserve the integrity of nature without damaging it. Effectively, this means that we should always buy organically certified or sustainably harvested ingredients. Protecting nature protects us all and furthers our relationship with our global health.

THE BEST SUPERFOODS

"Superfoods" are the perfect example of nature's incredible vitality. The classification is used to describe foods that are nutrient-rich, with a higher-than-average phytochemical profile, making them an invaluable addition to your diet. Research shows that when we take these superfoods in combination we get enhanced effects. For further details of individual foods, *see* The Pukka Pantry.

Berries Colorful berry fruits, such as blueberries, bilberries, raspberries, elderberries, and goji berries, are among the best cell-nourishing and -protecting foods available, as they are high in vitamins, phytonutrients, and phenolic compounds such as anthocyanins (which give the fruits their red or purplish color). They slow the reproduction of rogue cells and immobilize mutated cells, which helps us to age gracefully and healthfully and remain vital. Their juice reduces platelet levels, which decreases the risk of blood clots and offers circulatory system support. They also contain compounds that help to reduce inflammation and strengthen the body's collagen tissue. More specifically, they promote higher levels of "happy" HDL cholesterol and inhibit oxidation of "lousy" LDL cholesterol. Eat when in season on a daily basis.

Broccoli sprouts The sprouts from the broccoli plant contain some of the potent glucosinolates, including sulforophane, which is a cellular protector. Sprouts are therefore considered to delay aging and prevent degenerative diseases such as cancer. They also improve detoxification, which leads to benefits for many organs in the body, including the lungs, bowel, liver, bladder, breasts, and ovaries. Eat plentifully throughout the year.

Chlorella A microscopic algae, chlorella cleanses, alkalizes and protects the body, with a special focus on supporting immunity. It is one of the most nutritionally dense foods in the world, filled with antioxidants, amino acids, proteins, essential fatty acids, vitamins, minerals, and nucleic acids. It also has the highest-known concentration (three percent) of chlorophyll (*see* p.185) of any plant—just ⅛ ounce of chlorella provides the same amount of chlorophyll as 3½ ounces of raw spinach. Its health benefits include reducing cholesterol, healing wounds, regulating weight, balancing blood-sugar levels, improving digestion and reducing candida and inflammation. Specifically, its tough cell wall binds with heavy metals, pesticides and carcinogens, drawing them out from the body, making it a powerful detoxifier.

Flower pollen Collected by bees from plants, flower pollen is considered to be one of the most nutritious foods available, packed with proteins, vitamins, minerals, and amino acids. It strengthens the whole body and increases resistance to infections, and is a nerve tonic and energizing essence that improves both physical and intellectual performance. Although pollen appears to be unlimited, bee populations are now under threat, so check it comes from a sustainable source.

Spirulina Its name comes from its spiral structure and it is also known as a blue-green alga (even though it is not part of the algae species!), because of its pigment, phycocyanin, a powerful antioxidant. Its nutritionally dense composition makes spirulina useful for correcting nutritional deficiencies, replenishing amino acid and protein levels, building energy, enhancing endurance, nourishing blood, healing digestion, reducing candida, assisting nerve regeneration, building immunity, regulating weight, balancing blood-sugar levels, improving joint function, and reducing inflammation. It is specifically helpful in degenerative diseases.

Wheatgrass juice One of nature's most potent cellular and whole-body detoxifiers and rejuvenators, wheatgrass juice simultaneously cleanses and rebuilds. This is of special importance for slowing aging, preventing degenerative disease, optimizing athletic performance, and staying in peak mental condition. Wheatgrass juice is also specifically used for alleviating the symptoms of iron deficiency, suppurating wounds, intestinal inflammation, constipation, and ulcerative colitis, and cancer of the liver. Use cold-pressed when possible, to retain the delicate enzymes and nutrients.

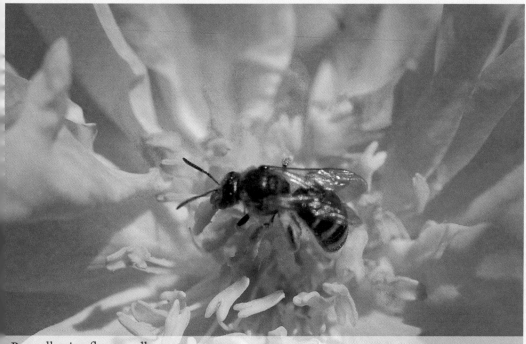

Bee collecting flower pollen

GAIA, GREED, AND ECOLOGY

Looking at health in the context of ecology rather than the usual medical paradigm can give us some useful insights. After all, this approach is an extension of the central Ayurvedic principle that everything is part of a whole. As human and environmental health involve working with each other to create harmony, we need always to consider them together.

Our planet as Gaia

The idea of the integrated nature of our own health and that of our world is expounded in what is known as Gaia Theory. Gaia is the name for the ancient Greek Earth goddess, sometimes called Mother Earth, and is the personification of nurture, care, and motherly love. The idea of the Earth and everything in it being one whole took on a deep ecological significance when, in the early 1970s, the scientist James Lovelock proposed his Gaia hypothesis. His idea is that the Earth is a single organism, with the biosphere, atmosphere, and the physical earth all interacting in a complex dynamic. Each of these components is communicating with the others through intricate feedback mechanisms in order to maintain the optimum conditions for life to exist. The value of this perspective is immense: it changes our whole world view from one of separation to one of inclusion.

We are a part of the Earth's being, just as the Earth is a part of ours. And we are perhaps Gaia's finest creation, with our ability to be conscious, to reason, and to communicate. But we might also be her greatest scourge as we selfishly pillage the Earth, polluting our life-giving water and air. This could be our greatest evolutionary mistake, as Gaia will dictate the rules of ecology without asking us for our opinion or even caring for our survival. She is interested in the whole, not only the part. Our resistance to considering the whole is challenging the normal homeostatic boundaries of the Earth's health, just as our modern lifestyles are pushing the limits of our own well-being.

Plundering the Earth

The resources of the world are finite. This is at odds with the idea of continuous exponential growth that contemporary economists and politicians seem to promise. Over the last 200 years the world's population has grown six times, but the economy has expanded a massive 68 times. If this rate of growth continues, by 2100 our economy will be 80 times bigger than it was in 1950. And while the needs of a growing population have always been a little beyond what the Earth can provide, it now looks as though we may well reach the limit of the Earth's resources.

Discussions of when we reach (or have reached) the point of "Peak Oil" (the point of maximum oil production after which extraction descends into continual decline) are continuing at a time when global emissions have risen by 40 percent since 1990. The Intergovernmental Panel on Climate Change has recommended that carbon emissions are limited to 450 parts per million in order to keep the average global temperature increase below 2°C (the level considered necessary to avoid dangerous climate change). This means that we need to reduce emissions to 15 percent below the 1990 total.

Health and ecology

Much work on the connection between human and planetary ecological health has been undertaken by herbalist David Hoffmann (director of the California School of Herbal Studies and former president of the American Herbalist Guild) and it is worth looking at this in some detail. His theory has four principle tenets. The first states that health is an expression of balance: inner homeostasis is a reflection of the planetary homeostasis, and *vice versa*. It is an extension of Lovelock's theory, which views the Earth as a self-regulating organism. The individual parts of the Earth's evolving biosphere are in a continual state of dialogue: the atmosphere, the ice caps, the rainforests, the mountain, and the seas communicate with each other all of the time. Any imbalance in either our inner environment or the outer environment upsets the other.

Hoffmann considers that human health is ecological relationship in action. All ecology is about relationship. In order to ensure health, the nature of the relationship, as well as the needs of both sides of the relationship, must be identified and understood. Because this relationship is in continual dynamic flux, it requires continual effort to find balance. It can be helpful to understand health as a dynamic movement toward this balance. If you are balanced you can only move out of balance.

Furthermore, health is an ecological bridge between our inner and outer worlds. How the edges of every organism engage with the perimeters of the next has a huge influence on our health and nature's health. From how our lungs engage with the air we breathe, to how our digestion manages the challenge of the foods we eat, from how our skin relates to the environment it touches, to how our senses experience and interpret the world—all appear to be critical to our health. What we let across our boundary and what we don't is essential to our future survival. And this situation is mirrored in nature as land meets sea, earth meets sky, desert meets savannah, and countryside meets city. These crossroads create a dynamic relationship between different phases in the ecological balance. They allow for change and adaptation but also create vulnerability.

Hoffmann's final tenet is that health and ecology are ultimately an expression of relationship. The very nature of relationship plays a role in human well-being and ecological balance. So, to be truly healthy, you need to explore your world, and your relationship with it, on all levels: from your attitude to your body, your connection with your diet, your relationship with your family to your experience of nature, and your intimacy with your spiritual life.

This world view, as outlined by both Lovelock and Hoffmann, emphasizes that our personal health must be addressed from many angles, and certainly in the context of the world in which we live. It is a distillation of all the great herbal medicine traditions and the essence with which I try to engage my patients. Understanding the interconnected nature of life is what fills my daily routines, work, and relationships. If anything is not contributing to the "whole" then it needs attention and a decision as to whether it should be let go or more closely nurtured. After all, true healing is about how we feel within our world as much as how we feel within ourselves; there is no separation between our nature and big Nature.

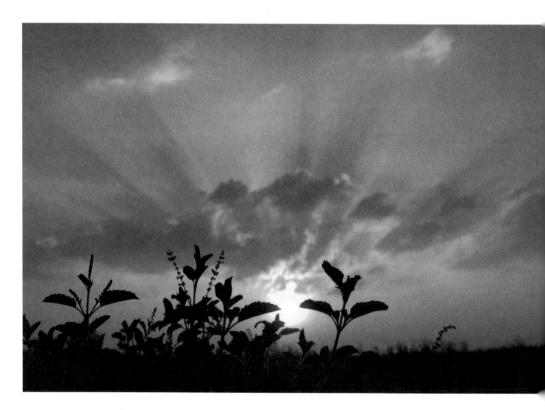

CONNECTING WITH NATURE

Nature brings us back to wholeness, reminding us of how we are part of a greater reality than just our individual selves. When we're feeling out of sorts, reconnecting with nature is one of the best ways to replenish. Conversely, being "disconnected" is the root cause of so many of the issues we face today. From the pervasive use of processed foods, through the destruction of precious forests, to widespread pollution, we are part of a society that is becoming more and more removed from the source of our sustenance. This separation is fueled by an assumption that we can take—and keep taking—without giving back.

On an individual level we've carved out a lifestyle that avoids the ebb and flow of nature's tides: eating food out of season, turning night into day, forever trying to hold on to youth. We've created a barrier between ourselves and our ecology, losing access to the rhythm of life and the wisdom that comes with it. Adrift, we float from one moment to the next. But it is possible to reconnect. Open your eyes to the magic before you: the first rays of dawn, the leaves in fall, running water. Cultivate a sensitivity to the world around you. Be present and aware of each sound, touch, sight, smell, and taste. This will allow you to be here in this moment, and that is a true connection with nature and with yourself. There are a number of ways in which we can truly connect with nature's mood, feeling, and cycles. Following a different lifestyle in each season can be very effective (*see Pukka Practice*, p.198), as are breathing practices, walking, and gardening.

Breathing

A simple and immediate way to connect with nature is through the breath. Like a spider's thread it weaves a path between our unconscious and conscious worlds, linking the inner and the outer, with each affecting the other. On the most literal, biological level, we know that we are connected through the processes of respiration and photosynthesis: plants release oxygen, which we breathe in; we exhale carbon dioxide, which plants absorb. Becoming aware of the usually subconscious process of breathing allows us to become present in the moment. When we forget the breath we forget ourselves; when we remember the breath we remember how we are part of a greater whole. Try it now.

Take a breath, deepen the inhalation, push it into your belly, let it rise in your chest, and then let out a long exhalation. Let it all go. How do you feel? Back in your body, connected with your present world? Well, that is where you belong.

You can do this anywhere, anytime, and if you forget, just start again, making this "return to breath" a part of your everyday practice to connect with nature.

✸ Walking

Walking links us to the Earth: with each stride we are in touch with the land. Connection is a two-way process: us to the Earth and the Earth to us, wind in hair, breath inside and out, with freedom all around. If ever there were a cure for a heavy mood it is a good walk, bringing into perspective how huge our world is, how awesome nature is, how remarkable our cities are, and how small and yet incredible we are.

For a deeper connection with nature, try a simple walking meditation. With every step become aware of your feet touching the ground. Feel the earth supporting you as your weight sinks down. As you move, notice all the muscles and the coordination involved in taking a step; feel your breath moving in and out with each stride; become aware of what your eyes can see. Carry on deepening this awareness: earth-feet-body-breath-earth-feet-body-breath. Soon you will become aware of your connection with nature: the space you are in and the space you are on. Now stop and stand still for a few moments, noticing how you have become one with the here and now.

✸ Gardening

If you don't have a space to garden, get one: an allotment, a land share, or even some pots on a windowsill. Gardening is easy and fun, and you can grow delicious foods, inspirational flowers, and healing herbs. Through some special magic, getting your hands dirty and caring for the soil will connect you with the rhythms of nature.

Planting seeds Many of the culinary herbs, such as basil, cilantro or parsley, are easy to grow. If you want to try something floral, chamomile, calendula (marigold), or geraniums are fun, delicious, and colorful. First find some good organic compost, a seed tray, and some seeds. Fill the seed tray with compost up to ½ inch from the top, pat it down, and sprinkle the seeds over the soil as evenly as possible. Cover with a little more compost, water lightly, and lay a sheet of glass or a plastic bag over the top of the tray to retain moisture and heat. Position the tray in a warm location and let nature work her magic. When the seeds have sprouted, transfer the individual seedlings into smaller containers.

SEASONAL LIFESTYLES

As we know, the climate in which we live intimately affects our health, due to the varying qualities of cooling, heating, dryness, or dampness that we experience. These qualities also affect the "taste" of the air, food, and water and our "feeling" of life. Different climate zones have their own patterns: Alaska is cold and dry; the Amazon hot and damp; the Sahara Desert hot and dry. The environment is, of course, always changing and so we need to keep our health in tune by adapting our lifestyle accordingly.

The best way to understand seasonal patterns is to observe the world around you. Take a look at your immediate environment: is it cold, hot, dry, or damp? Once you begin thinking along these lines you can see how this correlates with the Ayurvedic approach, through which it is possible to counteract the effects that the changing seasons can have on your health.

Staying healthy through the changing seasons means staying one step ahead: reducing the quality now that will be imbalanced in the next season. Follow a *pitta*, heat-reducing diet in early spring before it becomes aggravated in late spring, with symptoms of spring fevers and hay fever. Follow a *vata*, dryness-reducing diet in the summer to avoid fall, dry skin, eczema, dry coughs, and poor sleep. Follow a *kapha*, dampness-reducing diet in the winter before it appears as spring colds and allergies. For details of all of the above diets, *see* Nourishment, p.64.

THE EFFECTS OF THE SEASONS IN NORTHERN EUROPE

Season	Accumulating	Aggravating	Treatment
Early spring	*Pitta*, heat	*Kapha*, dampness	Reduce heat and dampness
Late spring	*Pitta*, heat	*Pitta*, heat	Reduce heat
Summer	*Vata*, dryness	*Pitta*, heat	Reduce heat and dryness
Early fall	*Vata*, dryness	*Vata*, dryness and cold	Reduce dryness
Late fall	*Kapha*, dampness	*Vata*, dryness and cold	Reduce dryness and cold
Winter	*Kapha*, dampness and cold	*Kapha*, dampness	Reduce dampness and cold

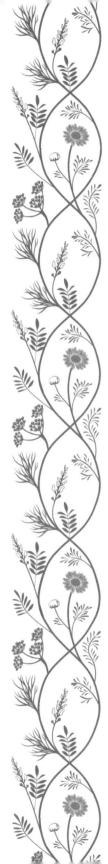

PUKKA PRACTICE

SEASONAL ROUTINES

When trying to align ourselves with the changing seasons we need to bear in mind the great Ayurvedic principle of "like increasing like" (*see* Constitution, p.14). To help keep you balanced, you need a diet and lifestyle that is opposite to the quality of the season (*see* the chart, previous page): cleansing in spring; cool in summer; oily in the fall; and warm in winter. If you are a mixed constitutional type, follow the advice in Constitution, *Pukka Practice*, p.33.

Spring routine

Spring is a time of growth, ascendancy, and new potential, with increased warmth and wetness from a thawing of the congealed damp of winter. By spring, because of the highly cold and wet qualities of winter and our heavier diet, *kapha* has accumulated and needs to be eliminated. Just as there are spring floods, with rivers overflowing, so there are internal "floods": the increased heat "melts" this *kapha* accumulation, causing spring colds and hay fever. While *vata* types like spring, if you have any problems associated with *vata* then this is the time to find balance. *Pitta* is balanced in the early part of spring, but can accumulate as the warmth increases later in the season. However, as *kapha* imbalances are the main threat, your spring routine should include some *kapha*-reducing habits.

Wake with the dawn and make the most of seasonal vitality. Sleeping in beyond 7am. aggravates *kapha*, so rise early to feel less tired, lazy, mucus-laden, and muzzy-headed.

Brush your teeth with a toothpaste containing fennel and clean your tongue with a tongue scraper.

Treat yourself to an oil massage using organic sesame or sunflower oil to revitalize your skin. Then have a hot shower to refresh your whole body.

Vigorous skin rubbing can be very valuable at this time for stimulating lymphatic circulation. Using your hands, start rubbing the feet and legs, progress to the arms and back and then to the chest and abdomen. This brings lymphatic fluid back to the heart, from where any toxins it has been carrying can be transported via the blood to the liver and kidneys for elimination.

Dry massage using herbal powder is also useful for regulating the lymphatic system, and for clearing fluid accumulation and cellulite from the skin. If you have fluid retention, Ayurveda recommends using chickpea flour or amla as a body rub. Having a sauna during the early part of spring will help to dry the excessive excretions that may occur at this time.

Make your first drink of the day a cup of hot ginger and lemon water to stimulate your digestion and cut through any mucus. Slice or grate ½-inch of fresh ginger into the cup, add hot water, and let infuse for a few minutes, before adding a squeeze of lemon with some honey.

Your yoga practice can include *kapha*-regulating postures that are dynamic, expansive, and stimulating (*see* Strength and Stillness, p.159). Practice some invigorating "brain-cleansing" breaths (*kapalabhati*—*see* Cleansing, p.88) after your postures.

Meals should be warm, light, and easy to digest. Emphasize bitter, pungent, and astringent foods, such as asparagus, spices, and beans, which will help to clear mucus and excess moisture toxins from the body. Increase light grains, such as rice, quinoa, barley, millet, and corn. Avoid concentrated sweet, sour, and salty flavors that are heavy and cause water retention. Honey (considered to be slightly astringent and warming) is the only sweetener *kapha* should have, as it helps to clear mucus.

Avoid ice, refrigerated foods eaten cold, eating too much, eating between meals, and sleeping in the day, as they will offset all of the other good work that you are doing. Help your body's natural efforts to find balance by supporting the seasonal clearing of the lungs using mild expectorants, such as pippali (*see* The Pukka Pantry) every day. Spring is a good time of year to cleanse your system of some of the accumulations of the winter months (*see* Cleansing, *Pukka Practice*, p.96).

Yellow flowers dominate in the spring and the "doctrine of signatures" (the idea that God has laid a signature over the Earth to guide us to which herbs are good for which diseases) says that yellow connects to the liver. After your initial course of *kapha*-clearing, move toward cleansing the liver of fatty and hot *pitta* accumulations by using some bitter herbs like yellow-flowering dandelion or neem. In late spring, turmeric (½ teaspoon) can be taken a couple of times a day with aloe vera juice to clear any latent heat and rejuvenate the liver.

Go to bed before 11pm to ensure that you get adequate rest to wake up before 7am.

Summer routine

In summer the Fire element is higher: there is more warmth, dryness, and lightness. These qualities increase *pitta* and, as the summer progresses, begin to aggravate *vata*. The increase in external environmental heat can displace the digestive fire (*agni*), which is drawn to the surface in inflammatory symptoms such as hay fever and prickly heat. Hence, summer is naturally a time of calming and reducing *pitta*.

In summer we tend to awaken earlier, so get up at the time you like with the morning sun.

Brush your teeth with a cooling toothpaste that includes neem or peppermint to clear *pitta* from the mouth.

Have a light massage using virgin coconut oil at room temperature to nourish and gently cool the skin. Wash it off with lukewarm water.

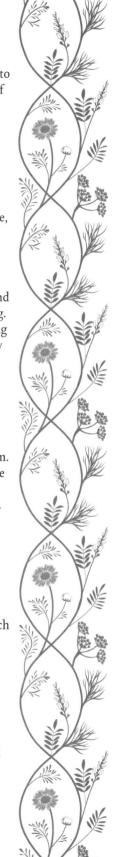

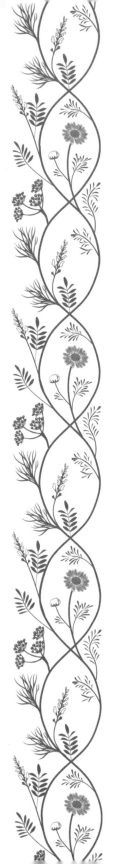

For a blissful start to your day, walk with bare feet on a cool, dewy lawn.

Begin your yoga practice with a calming breathing practice. If the temperature is extremely hot, then the "cooling breath" (*sheetali pranayama*) is most appropriate: roll your tongue into a tube and then draw the cool air in through this tube and out through your nostrils.

Because of the heat, *pitta* tends to build up in the digestive system in the summer. Yoga poses that feature abdominal stretches, twists, and internal massage (*see* Strength and Stillness, p.157) will help to clear *pitta* from its main site in the liver and small intestine; this will also help your eyes, which are energetically linked to the liver. Eye exercises (*see* Rejuvenation, p.112) relax the eyes and increase circulation, helping to carry away any irritating stress.

After yoga, anoint yourself with fragrant rose oil. Place a drop on your "third eye" (in between your eyebrows), throat, and navel to keep these centers of awareness cool, calm, and collected.

Your diet should consist of sweet, bitter, and astringent flavors, and be light and easy to digest. For breakfast include a nourishing drink, such as almond milk: soak ten almonds in water overnight; in the morning peel them, liquidize with warm milk (cows or rice), then add a pinch of saffron and a sweetener to taste. Try to eat lunch at around noon, when the sun is at its zenith. And then for supper enjoy a light meal of basmati rice, sprouted mung beans, and green leafy vegetables. If you are being strictly Ayurvedic, salad should be avoided at night so that your *vata* is not upset.

It is best to avoid all dark meats—beef, lamb, pork—as well as citrus fruits, tomato, garlic, onion, pungent flavors, and salt and sour dairy products, as these all increase *pitta*.

It may be useful to take aloe vera juice throughout the summer to clear *pitta* from the digestive system and soothe and replenish a hot body.

Drink energetically cooling herbal teas of peppermint, licorice, fennel, and roses. Or try rose syrup elixir: collect fresh rose petals in a glass and cover them in sugar overnight (leave in the moonlight for extra cooling effect). In the morning mix the syrup in your almond milk or dilute with water.

As the weather heats up it is very important to be on your guard for *pitta* emotions, such as irritation and anger. If you feel a bit "hot under the collar," a good trick is to take a large sip of water and hold it in your mouth. The water cools your *pitta* and keeps you quiet. I can tell you, it works!

Before bed, and especially if it has been a hot day, rub the soles of your feet with coconut or castor oil to draw all the heat down to your feet and away from your head so as to avoid headaches.

For pure indulgence, wash your face in organic rosewater and spray it in your bedroom. In pursuit of the perfectly balanced *pitta* home, fill your house and bedroom with fragrant roses, honeysuckle, and jasmine.

As *pitta* peaks at around midnight, it is really helpful to get to bed before 11pm.

Fall routine

The Air element is predominant in fall: more lightness, dryness (temporarily), coolness, the erratic "winds of change." These qualities in nature have a tendency to aggravate *vata*, which has already begun accumulating at the end of summer. As *vata* regulates the nervous system, the levels of moisture in the body, how relaxed we feel and how well we digest food, these can easily become unsettled. If our digestion is functioning below par then harmful *ama* (toxins) can also increase. Diseases where toxins and *vata* mix together, such as arthritis, can appear. To balance *vata*, limit exposure to cold winds and dryness and try to minimize erratic behavior. Toward the end of fall, when it is colder and wetter, *kapha* begins to accumulate, and in turn requires balancing.

Rise at 7am when the world is still and calm.

Brush your teeth with nourishing herbal toothpaste that includes gum-strengtheners such as licorice, haritaki, and mint.

A slightly quirky but nevertheless effective idea for balancing *vata* is to hold some warm sesame oil in your mouth for three minutes (use about ¼ cup). Although it sounds strange, it nourishes the mouth, strengthens the teeth, stops any bleeding, and prevents receding gums.

Massage yourself with warm sesame or *mahanarayan* oil, which offsets the seasonal tendency to dryness, cracking joints, and stiff muscles. After a warm shower, place a drop of *nasya* oil (*see* Constitution, p.27) in your nostrils and ears to offset the damaging effect of the elements.

Start your yoga practice with "alternate nostril breathing" (*nadi shodhana*) to eliminate the *vata* toxins that restrict your nervous system, circulation and subtle channels. *See* Strength and Stillness, p.162 for full instructions.

The yoga poses that regulate *vata* include the Wind-relieving pose (*pawan mukt asana*), all inverted poses where the head moves below the waist (e.g., Headstand, Shoulder Stand), all twists and slow Sun Salutations, with breaths in each posture (*see* Strength and Stillness, p.156).

Apply heavy scents, such as vetiver, patchouli, or a *vata* essential oil, on the "third eye" (eyebrow-center) and throat.

Your diet should comprise warm foods that are sweet, mildly spicy, sour and salty to increase moisture and help you feel nourished and grounded. Begin the day with a small bowl of oat, rice or quinoa oatmeal, which can be flavored with maple syrup or honey and cinnamon. For lunch and supper choose nourishing foods such as steamed vegetables, soup, or kicharee (for recipe *see* Cleansing, *Pukka Practice*, p.98). Avoid too much raw salad, cold drinks, ice, beans, fermented foods, and yeast, as they cause wind and may destabilize your digestion.

Take a teaspoon of chywanaprash in the morning to keep your energy and immunity intact. If you feel out of sorts, are not sleeping as well as you usually do, or are stressed, take ashwagandha as a replenishing tonic.

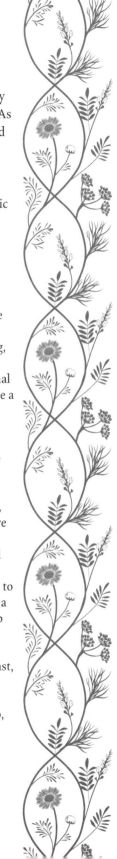

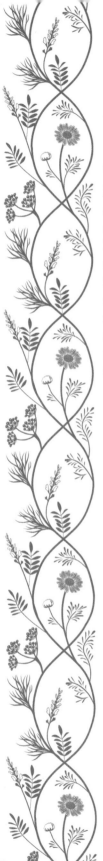

Early fall is a common time to perform a seasonal detoxification to prepare for the winter ahead (*see* Cleansing, *Pukka Practice*, p.96).

At the end of the day enjoy a delicious cup of milk simmered with a pinch of saffron, nutmeg, and cardamom, and settle in as early as possible for a blissful night's sleep.

Winter routine

During winter the Earth's energy is drawn back into herself. It is a time of rest, storing, and preparation. This is when you need to be more grounded, internalized and still. The weather is often cold, wet, cloudy, and heavy and is dominated by the Earth and Water elements. Because of the Ayurvedic rule that "like increases like," all these qualities aggravate *kapha*; remember that *kapha* means "that which flourishes in water." In climates where there is a long winter, this extended period of cold can cause *vata* to become out of kilter, and so people with *vata* imbalances really need to be mindful in these constitutionally identical conditions. If you have a *kapha* constitution you should follow as many of these recommendations as you can. If you are *vata* you will also benefit, but if you are *pitta* then keep clearing heat from the inside of your body while keeping the exterior warm.

Sleeping in until a bit later is fine in winter, as staying warm in your bed helps you to rejuvenate.

When you get up, brush your teeth with stimulating cinnamon, clove, and haritaki toothpaste to reduce sensitivity to the cold.

Holding warm sesame oil in the mouth (*see* Fall routine, previous page) is also useful in winter.

Massage yourself with warm sesame oil or *kapha* oil to offset the seasonal tendency to coldness, aching joints, and "frozen shoulder." Leave some time for the oil to be absorbed, then take a warm shower.

Put a drop of *nasya* oil in the nose (*see* Fall routine, previous page). This can help to alleviate depression and Seasonal Affective Disorder (SAD) by bringing lightness and clarity.

For your first drink of the day sip warm ginger water. Add a twist of lemon with some honey to help relax the digestive system, wake up your appetite, and encourage a healthy bowel motion.

Practice stimulating yoga to balance *kapha*, increase your circulation, and clear excess mucus. Do vigorous Sun Salutations (*surya namaskar*) until you are warm and your breathing becomes deep. Also include some strong backward and forward bends that open the chest and help move stagnant *kapha* (*see* Strength and Stillness, p.159.)

Your diet should comprise warm foods that are mildly spicy, slightly salty, and nourishing to clear *kapha* but not aggravate *vata*. We usually eat more in the winter because our digestive fire is stronger, as the cooler weather constricts the surface of the body, pushing the heat back to our core. A small bowl of warm oat, cornmeal (polenta), barley or rice oatmeal will set you up for a bracing day. Add cinnamon, cloves, and honey. Lunch and supper should be wholesome meals, avoiding too many cold, wet, and damp foods that are excessively sweet or taken straight from the refriderator. Barley is one of the best grains for *kapha*, as its drying quality gently clears fluids from the body and can refresh a sluggish digestion; it is also good for nourishing *vata*. Drink spicy teas throughout the day to stoke your inner fire.

Take a teaspoon of chywanaprash in the morning to keep your energy and immunity intact at this time of change. If you are easily disturbed by the cold,   wet, and heavy qualities of winter then you may benefit from taking trikatu as it will blow away any colds, coughs, poor circulation, and nasal drips.

Settle in for a relaxing evening. Ayurveda suggests that an occasional glass of warming wine may be beneficial in the winter to encourage circulation and stimulate digestion. Before bed, make a delicious glass of hot, spicy milk: nutmeg is calming and promotes sound sleep.

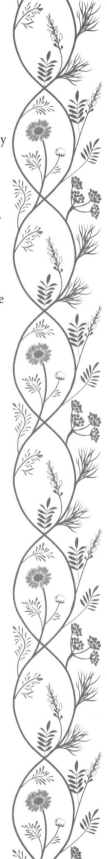

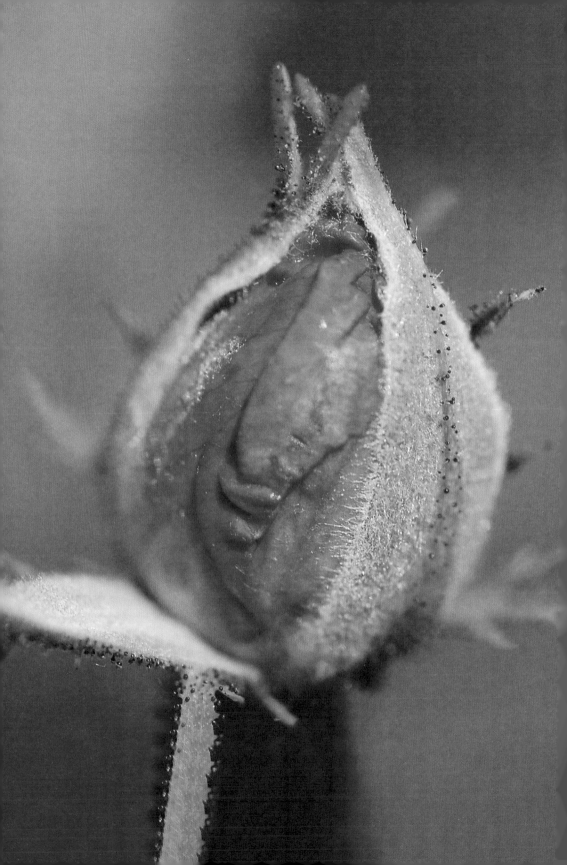

7 RELATIONSHIP

"One who sees equally the entire universe in his own self and his own self in the entire universe is in possession of true knowledge."

CHARAKA SAMHITA

All relationships are about love: an unconditional love and acceptance of your own pure perfection that shines into every relationship. Love is at the heart of the world, just as it is at the heart of your life. Your relationships with your lover, your family, your friends, and the world around you define the quality of your emotional wholeness and reflect your relationship with yourself. But there are many paths to tread on the journey toward the perfect relationship, toward an unconditional acceptance of yourself as an embodiment of perfect, divine, unconditional love. It requires deep awareness, persistence and, most importantly, compassion.

ME, MYSELF AND I

"*Through Love all that is bitter will sweeten.*
Through Love all that is copper will be gold.
Through Love all dregs will turn to purest wine.
Through Love all pain will turn to medicine.
Through Love the dead will all become alive.
Through Love the king will turn into a slave!"
MAWLANA JALAL-AL-DIN RUMI, 13TH-CENTURY POET AND SUFI MYSTIC

Traveling deep inside ourselves, traversing the dark, murky corners of our own pain and recognizing the inherent nature of our suffering is a well-trodden route to the highest peaks of inner vision and bliss. Fortunately, there are many helpers along the way. These are the people you meet every day, for they are also searching for this true experience of unconditional love. They are the reflective mirrors of our nearest and dearest, wise guardians in the form of old friends, spiritual guides, or teachers, who hold up the looking glass to our souls, revealing what we need to learn. As we embrace our passions and delve into the mystery of life, we unite with the majestic complexity of nature; and if we follow the signs, this can help us understand who we really are.

We need to tread softly with light steps and tender words, which can bring us to the place where we really always are: in the heart of love. A wise woman once told me to live "with an empty head and open heart." Although I often live with a busy head and veiled heart, when I tread softly I can much more easily return to this place of living with a loving heart.

CULTIVATING COMPASSION

"*Compassion is that which makes the heart of the good move at the pain of others. It crushes and destroys the pain of others; thus, it is called compassion. It is called compassion because it shelters and embraces the distressed.*"

THE BUDDHA, FROM THE DHAMMAPADA

If life is love then we need compassion, for those we know, for those we meet, and for every being in the world, because everyone wants to be content and happy, and yet everyone suffers. However, first we need compassion for ourselves, as only through understanding our own disconnection—our own "dis-ease"—can we touch the pain that needs healing. When you perceive the nature and cause of your own sorrows then you can recognize another's suffering more personally and truthfully. In Ayurveda the duty of a doctor is to be able "to enter the heart of the patient" and understand what they are truly feeling. You can develop this quality in all your relationships: ask yourself, "What is the feeling behind these words?" and, "What is the feeling behind this behavior?" Then you will know the truth.

The Dalai Lama says, "If you want others to be happy, practice compassion. If you want to be happy, practice compassion." The only way to do this is to integrate certain practices into your daily life: physical, mental, and emotional exercises that will help develop compassion, simple exercises that mark your intention to grow.

Massage

Out of all the practices that help us on this long journey, massage has to be the best, simply because it is a pure expression of love. Gentle, soothing, and loving, it is a fantastically relaxing way to become intimately acquainted. A central part of Ayurvedic living, it can be practiced by anyone. Giving yourself a massage can bring kindness into your life. As you knead your tensions, you honor your needs and yourself. As you touch your skin, you can shed your armor and heal your wounds. You can welcome self-healing and remember your wholeness. Rather like meditation, massage helps you to reintegrate. Of course, we usually think of massage as something we share with someone else and these same intentions can also be offered to them. *See also* Strength and Stillness, *Pukka Practice*, p.170.

Writing

Letting your mind flow with loving thoughts is an inspiring and intimate way to keep compassion close at heart. It is very opening and humbling to acknowledge pain, disappointments, desires, and feelings. By writing about the areas in your life that you find challenging you can identify a need for nurturing and, with your compassionate heart awakened, find ways to bring this nourishment into your life. It's a remarkable thing, but writing about the people, places, and things that you love and cry for can help identify what you are really feeling. Returning to a favorite Ayurvedic analogy, writing helps us digest our feelings by welcoming what is sustaining and releasing what is not.

 ## Contemplative meditation

Meditation is both the symbol and expression of our intention to grow. Sitting still, alone with our thoughts and feelings, we can honor missed opportunities, passing desires, remembered disappointments, as well as our inner strength, personal wisdom, and ability to forgive and love. There are a number of practices that you can include in your daily routine, all of which help to develop empathy, compassion, and understanding. They involve engaging your inner and self-reflecting "witness," emptying your head, and opening your heart. *See* p.210 for specific meditation practices.

The Metta Sutta

All of the practices listed below are embodied in The Metta Sutta, an ancient Buddhist poem about "loving-kindness." Loving-kindness is defined as the strong wish for the welfare and happiness of others. The poem is repeated as a study aid, to help generate the essence of loving-kindness within oneself and for all beings.

The Pali word *metta* is multidimensional, encompassing loving-kindness, amity, goodwill, benevolence, fellowship, concord, inoffensiveness, and nonviolence. Essentially *metta* is an altruistic attitude of deep love and friendliness, as distinguished from mere amiability based on self-interest. Or, as the contemporary Buddhist teacher Sogyal Rinpoche describes it succinctly: "Look after yourself so that you can look after others and look after others so that they can look after you."

An abbreviated version of The Metta Sutta can be learned by heart and used as part of your daily practice for yourself, your family, your community, and whomever else you hope to reach with a feeling of loving-kindness. Practicing it every day will generate healing energy and bring compassion into your life:

"May I feel safe and protected.
May I live in peace.
May I be free from suffering.
May I be happy."

The Metta Sutta:
the Buddha's words on loving-kindness

This is the work for those who are skilled and peaceful,
who seek the good:
May they be able and upright, straightforward,
of gentle speech and not proud.
May they be content and easily supported,
Unburdened with their senses calmed.
May they be wise, not arrogant
and without desire for the possessions of others.
May they do nothing mean or that the wise would reprove.

May all beings be happy. May they live in safety and joy.
All living beings, whether weak or strong,
tall, stout, medium, or short, seen or unseen,
Near or distant, born or to be born, may they all be happy.

Let no one deceive another or despise any being in any state,
Let none by anger or hatred wish harm to another.
As a mother watches over her child,
willing to risk her own life to protect her only child,
So with a boundless heart should one cherish all living beings,
Suffusing the whole world with unobstructed loving-kindness.

Standing or walking, sitting or lying down,
during all one's waking hours,
May one remain mindful of this heart
and this way of living that is the best in the world.
Unattached to speculations, views, and sense desires,
with clear vision,
Such a person will never be reborn in the cycles of suffering.

Distributed by the Chenrezig Project. *See* Resources p.251 for more details.

MEDITATION PRACTICES

The following meditations will help you cultivate compassion in order to experience more easily a state of loving-kindness.

Meditation on suffering

Settle your body, calm your breath, and allow your immediate thoughts to flow away down the river of your consciousness. Start to become aware of anything that is causing you pain in your life: sadness, confusion, tension. Conjure up a memory of an event or a person that brought you this experience of pain and notice how you feel as you remember. Is the pain located in a particular part of your body; what does it feel like; does it have a particular quality? Just sit with it as though you are watching from a short distance away; maybe the pain intensifies, softens, or dissolves. But, whatever happens in your meditation, know that this pain is true for you, and start to become aware of how you can be kind to yourself about this issue. It is your pain, but it is not you and you can choose how you care for it. As the petals of your heart unfurl, feel how you can hold, tend, and forgive yourself for this pain. Cradle it for a while and then let any thoughts and feeling of this pain pass as you float gently down the stream. And move on.

Think of someone you know and love. Imagine any suffering they experience and explore how this feels, how this hurts, where it hurts; feel the pain that your loved one feels. Now notice your feelings as your heart opens to their pain; how tender you feel for them; how accepting you are of their struggle. Let any frustrations, resentments, and anger bubble up – they may be real, too. And let them go. See an image of this person in your heart and bathe them, anoint them, soothe them. In your compassion you can know their suffering, honor and love them.

Now come back to your breath flowing quietly in and out, sense your body and the ground beneath you as you notice how you feel. Try and be with this feeling throughout your day.

Meditation on seeking happiness

In this wonderful practice you recognize that your needs and the needs of the person you are engaging with are exactly the same. Because it is internal and private you can very easily bring it into your everyday life, even if you're out and about. It's especially useful in "conflict" relationships where your wounds are easily opened and your intention for a positive outcome gets knocked off course by old and unconscious habits.

Whenever you feel it appropriate, repeat to yourself:

"Just like me, this person is seeking happiness in their life.
Just like me, this person is trying to avoid pain and suffering.
Just like me, this person has known sadness, grief, and loneliness.
Just like me, this person is seeking to learn about life and fulfill their needs."

As I seem to have the emotional memory of a goldfish, persistently forgetting to live in this way, I write myself notes to help me remember this.

Meditation on releasing suffering

Sit in any comfortable position and close your eyes. Let your breath settle into a gentle rhythm and come to the present moment.

Think of any person you know who is suffering. Experience their pain. Know how it feels when you are suffering and how it can hold you back. Imagine that you are watching them from above. Notice how you feel as you see them suffer. Then wish them to be free of it. Watch them flower as their pain leaves.

As you become comfortable with this practice, try focusing on someone who has upset you. Hold an image of them in your mind's eye. Remember what you experienced them doing to you and how you felt. Think about that person, their life, their situation. What was their childhood like; how did their parents treat them; where do they live; who are their friends; what are their aspirations? Try to understand the level of suffering that the person was in to have made them behave in such a way toward you. How upset or disturbed must they be to have done that to you? Feel their pain. Understand that their actions are not because of you, but have come from their suffering.

At this point you could repeat the words from the happiness meditation, above.

Now imagine how you can be with this person when you next meet. How will you feel about them? How can you help them feel safe? Now that you have developed some 'space' around the situation that created this problem, notice how you feel. Experience the compassion you feel for that person. When you are ready, feel the problem dissolve and the love emerge.

Now come back to your awareness of where you are and how you are feeling. Open your eyes and return to your day with a deeper understanding of your intention of living with compassion.

ILLNESS AS A SYMBOL

"That person who always eats wholesome food, enjoys a regular lifestyle, remains unattached to the objects of the senses, gives and forgives, loves truth, and serves others is without disease."

ASHTANGA HRIDAYA SAMHITA

Our illness can be our teacher. If you can get "under the skin" of your "dis-ease," you can gain deep insights into why you are unbalanced, which in turn can guide you to changing the patterns that are leading to this state—illness is really a symbol of what is unbalanced. If we listen then we can understand ourselves more and we might even get better. To give an oversimplified example, if you get a tummy upset, is it because you ate too many doughnuts or because you are intolerant to wheat? And did you eat too many doughnuts because you feel insecure and unloved and the doughnuts were an easy, temporary fix? Or have you become intolerant to wheat because you keep overeating doughnuts? Is there something more nourishing you can do?

In Ayurveda different organs and parts of your body are related to different emotions:

Liver Held emotions, frustration, *pitta*
Lungs Held grief, sadness, *kapha*
Kidneys Held fear, anxiety, *vata*
Heart Unbalanced joy, unbalanced anger
Digestion Lack of nourishment, lack of love
Eyes Connect with liver, anger, *pitta*
Ears Connect with kidneys, fear, *vata*
Nose Connects with lungs, grief, *kapha*
Skin Connects with heart, nervous system, anxiety

If you have an imbalance in any of these areas in the body you can look at your relationship with those emotions. Not every liver imbalance will be because you are frustrated, but seen in context, liver imbalances do lead to a tendency toward this state. Although we all have some aspects of each of these emotions, one or two tend to predominate both constitutionally and at different stages of our life. If a particular health imbalance keeps cropping up, it is worth using these simple analogies to explore what your illness symbolizes for you.

LIVING FROM THE HEART

"*You are never given a wish without also being given the power to make it true. You may have to work for it, however.*"
RICHARD BACH, WRITER

Every experience needs digestion and assimilation. If our emotional *agni*, the digestive fire of our heart, is depleted for any reason, then highly emotional experiences will be more difficult to work through. To keep your heart's fire burning it needs to be nourished. If you are aware of your heart's needs then it burns more brightly; meditation helps this, as does writing a journal or speaking to a friend or counselor. Some of the best ways to live from the heart come from these shared experiences.

Positive relationships are obviously essential to our happiness. Studies show that a supportive social network and positive relationships with partners, carers, teachers, and coworkers result in physical and emotional healing, happiness, and life satisfaction, and prevents isolation and loneliness, which are major factors in depressive illness. But we have to learn how to create relationships that meet our needs. This may be finding a safe, supportive, and nonjudgmental self-help group to help us with any traumas. A supportive group of friends or a good relationship with a counseling therapist or healing practitioner can be really helpful. We also need to learn techniques that boost self-esteem and a sense of inner confidence: spending time in nature helps us connect with the world around us; taking moderate exercise and walking in the open air alleviate depression; finding a sense of purpose that can be shared with your community creates a sense of belonging; developing a self-supporting daily practice such as yoga, meditation, or prayer can instill spiritual values that give your journey roots and strength.

"*The beauty of the heart is the lasting beauty: its lips give to drink of the water of life. Truly it is the water, that which pours, and the one who drinks. All three become one when your talisman is shattered. That oneness you can't know by reasoning.*"
RUMI, FROM *MATHNAWI*, BOOK II

If you can incorporate some of these skills into your life, then you can tenderly touch your heart and open those areas with which you feel uncomfortable. You can nurture your pain and release the suffering.

PUKKA PERSPECTIVES

EAST OR WEST: WHICH WAY TO NIRVANA?

We all want to be happy. Our modern world reflects this aspiration in advertising, the media, celebrity, and fashion, but it seems clear that none of these is the true route to happiness. So where can it be found? We live at a unique time in history when improvements in communication mean that it is easy to learn from the methods and values that different cultures have adopted to experience happiness. True happiness is often expressed in Indian religions by the term "Nirvana," which literally means "without wind." This refers to the enlightened state of being whereby you are no longer blown about by the "winds" of *karma*, rebirth, greed, hate, or delusion. It implies a perfect state of being: at peace and full of compassion. Can the philosophies and practices of the East and West, embodied respectively in the traditions of self-realization and psychotherapy, help us find Nirvana?

The self-realization of the East

The Eastern approach to finding happiness is, generally speaking, through techniques that lead to the realization of our true nature as "pure consciousness." In broad terms, pure consciousness is a state of being that transcends our usual identification with our name, body, and mind to one of integration, of oneness with our self, and the universal spirit. Indian tradition teaches that one way to get nearer to this experience of knowing who I am, to experiencing oneness, is to practice the repetition of *neti neti*, or "I am not this, I am not that." For example, "I am not really Sebastian, that is just the name for this body and character; I am not my body, it is just a transient mass of protein, fats, and carbohydrates; I am not my thoughts, they are a continual flux of impressions, desires, and aversions." All I am left with is the reality of being pure consciousness, pure bliss.

When we become integrated with the entire continuum of universal awareness we become one whole as opposed to one individual. The sun is the light in our mind; the wind is our breath; the sea is the water running

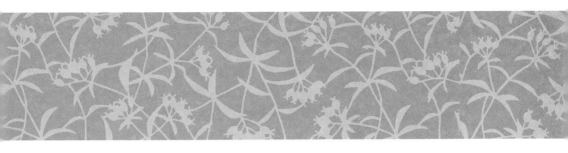

in our veins; the earth is our body. Suddenly everything is one. Your heart opens, the whole cosmos rushes in, billions of galaxies orbit within you and, unthinkingly, you experience a cosmic bliss of oneness that exists as one truth for ever.

Depending on your teacher and tradition, the path to this happiness, or Nirvana, could involve meditation, bodily purification, physical exercises, intellectual development, devotion, and direct perception (the Zen Buddhist technique of using *koans*—poems and stories—to help bypass the rational mind and access the intuition). By all accounts it's a long path, requiring lots of effort to prepare you. Take yoga, which literally means "to yoke," as two oxen might be joined together, creating an analogy of the union between our inner spirit and universal consciousness. Practicing yoga seriously is as hard as plowing a field with your bare hands to prepare the ground for the planting of seeds. Germination is inherent within the seed, just as being pure consciousness is inherent within you. Unifying your heart and mind, body, and soul, consciousness with pure consciousness, sounds like hard work but, ultimately, it is a state of effortless being. We can be it; we cannot try to be it.

This awareness of self-realization is not about an intellectual understanding of our union with universal consciousness but a direct experience of it, right now—BANG, like a flash of light! As Ken Wilber teaches, it is not the water or the waves but the wetness; this freedom has no form, no limit, no goal. You do not see anything when you experience pure consciousness; you become *everything*. As pure consciousness is always free and can never be contained, any belief that limits this realization will lead us away from happiness. Like the clear blue sky, universal consciousness is a pure and limitless expanse of open oneness. Any feelings of anger, sadness, or greed that obstruct this experience of oneness lead to unhappiness and are completely illusory. They exist in our mind due to a past experience, and are really like clouds floating through the sky. They are only problems because we hold on to and identify with them as problems.

The solution that the East teaches is to exist as a "witness," to observe the fluctuations and vagaries of life emerging and dissolving in each moment. We do not need to own them or let them go, for they are never ours—we just watch them flow by. Indian spiritual teachings are full of metaphors that illuminate our illusory and transient identification with our experiences in life: mistaking a stick lying by the side of the road for a snake; the way salt dissolves in water so that we can't see it, and so on. They all point to how we confuse what is not real for reality, when all we need to do is see reality as it is: here and now, the eternal bliss of oneness.

Psychotherapy in the West

By contrast, psychotherapy is based on that the belief that happiness comes from uprooting the conditioning that makes a person unhappy. In the pursuit of self-knowledge, the focus is on becoming aware of the pattern that has led to the problem. Taking the lead from the client, the psychotherapist will pursue the client's perceived shortcomings in order to help them become what they would like to become.

Many different fields of psychotherapy have been developed in the West over the past century, although they are all based on the nature of your relationships with yourself and the world around you. This idea of interconnection is clearly defined by the founders of the Gestalt movement of psychotherapy: "It is meaningless to define a breather without air, a walker without gravity and ground, an irascible without obstacles, and so on for every animal function." Another common thread is the tendency to examine the experience of relationship by exploring loneliness. By taking us on a journey through our life, therapy seeks to help the person identify why they feel alone, where the pattern began, and when it is repeated. Because we live in relationships with our family, sexuality, society, and culture, this often involves a detailed investigation into how we engage with these formative life experiences.

The intention is for the parts of us exposed by this exploration to be reintegrated so we become present and whole. By becoming aware of those

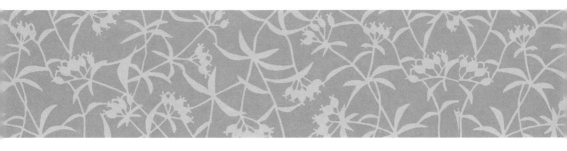

fragmented patterns and habits that no longer serve us—the overpowering feelings of rejection, fear, and worthlessness that we learn as children— they can be consciously rediscovered. The suppressed can safely resurface. We can be an adult, equal with our boss, partner, or our parents. We can be a powerful guide for our children and a compassionate lover with our beloved. Our lonely "littleness" does not need to dominate our relationships reactively. With the attentive guidance of the "witnessing" therapist, our conditioning can be unfurled to reveal the heart behind our protective armor. The "inner critic" can be silenced and we can relearn who we really are, and to feel and express what we really experience. We learn to give to ourselves the acceptance we sought as a child from our family.

Reaching Nirvana

As they say in India, there are many paths to the top of the mountain, but the view from the summit is always the same. Ultimately, successful psychotherapy and self-realization both lead us to a similar place: to our primordial birthright of unconditional love. The welcoming in of unconditional self-love enables you to unconditionally love others. Because our attitude to the outside world is purely a reflection of our attitude to our internal musings, our entire relationship with life can blossom. The reintegration of pain creates a field of love.

Self-realization seeks awakening through integration of universal consciousness; psychotherapy through integration of internal consciousness. But perhaps they are the same thing. While some forms of psychotherapy merely change a behavior pattern or enable contentment in your situation, the ability of therapy to highlight internal shadows can be very useful on the path to self-realization. There are so many obstacles to seeing the reality of life, so many chances to trip up on the path of living in unconditional love, that each approach serves the other. Psychotherapy serves the suppressed, the repressed, the hidden, in order to reveal what is really there; self-realization serves the ever-present, the all-pervasive, the all-powerful, in order to help us let go of pain. Both, especially when practiced together, can solve the condition of suffering and offer you the ocean of love.

LOVE

Experiencing love is the wellspring of our life. From this fountain of inspiration we can swim into the world and flourish as individuals. And we each have our own style and methods for trying to flourish in love: it is an especially personal path that we tread to togetherness. When so many relationships end in pain, frustration, and disappointment, sometimes we can lose sight of why we seek them. It is because relationships bring us support, friendship, intimacy, and love; they bring us to life. All of these ideas work for all relationships—family, children, friends—but here I'd like to focus on our amorous partnerships.

Love relationships bring us the opportunity for incredible transformation where we can find our sense of the beloved within ourselves through communion with someone else. We could choose to live our lives in isolation and deny these needs, or exist in relationships that require compromises—but we want (and deserve) more. We want communion, growth, passion, sharing, and unity. And this requires courage, openness, and patience with ourselves and with our partners. It may seem ironic, but to love another truly we need to love ourselves.

Vulnerability

A true relationship creates a space in which those parts of us that have been shut away can creep out and see the light again. It allows us the opportunity to grow. But that potential for change requires us to expose the most sensitive parts of our hearts: our fears, jealousies, rage, sense of worthlessness. This takes us to the edge of our comfort zone and exposes our frailties. But it is the pain of loneliness and exposure that helps us to seek deeper levels of intimacy and love. This is challenging work, because in an honest relationship we are faced with a mirror that regularly confronts us with our vulnerabilities. We have the choice, moment to moment, to dive into the whirlpool of our fears that potentially leads us to love, or to run away, tail between legs, to come across the same problems again.

Intellectually, being loving sounds very easy, but if your heart is anything like mine, emotional maturity is not always there when you want it. We revert to our own default patterns of behavior, which can often be childish. In any long-term relationship, as we move from the first impulses of romantic passion into everyday life, we have to face ourselves and all our old familiar demons yet again; as they say in Zen Buddhism, "After the ecstasy, the laundry." Because the love we have for ourselves is inextricably intertwined with the love we have for others we have to stay conscious with what type of love we are really offering: is it selfless and unconditional or needy and greedy? It usually takes time to change and we have to listen, appreciate, support, and share our feelings and awareness with our love partner, and with an open heart. Otherwise we will end up compromising, which never makes anyone happy or loving, but pushes our dreams away and increases our frustrations because our truth is not honored. Unchosen compromise shuts us down, little by little, until eventually we close. It's another form of death.

Rediscovering you

The paradox is that we want love but don't know how to receive or give it truly. Few of us enter relationships with high self-esteem, so we are confused both when love is offered and when given the opportunity to love. Over the years we have all compromised with ourselves in order to be loved. However loving our upbringing has been, we end up with the experience of separation from love, whether at birth from our mother's enwombed love, or the separation we perceive from not fulfilling our parents' expectations, or even the separation from God's love.

As we try to fit into our unintelligible world we conform, and as we conform we stop being ourselves, and then we stop liking ourselves—we have compromised. In a sense, the path of adulthood is the journey of rediscovering who we really are by healing the wounds inflicted by these concessions to survival. A loving relationship is a perfect place to help heal these wounds. But, as they are exposed, it can be hard not to recoil and try to protect yourself. Just think of the last time you were defensive or aggressive with your partner: was it really as a result of what they were doing or were you trying to protect something? To find deep love we need to find boundless mercy for our perceived shortcomings. Perhaps it is even our life's work really to love our body, our mind, and our spirit: who we really are, just as we are.

Loving support

One of the best supports on this path to rebuilding self-esteem is our friends. They can help reflect your transformations and remind you of your inherent beauty. In this context a friend may be someone you trust, or it may be a lover, a counselor or therapy group—even all three. It is essential that you build a support network of friends, whoever they may be, who can help remind you of your true self.

I think it is our love of pure consciousness, which some may call Spirit, that is really expressed in a love relationship. Because Spirit is so subtle and so sensitive, it relates to our experience of touch. As we close our eyes we can imagine we are a part of a vast expanse of greatness, of light and majesty. If we do not feel good enough ourselves how can we partake in this spacious divinity? When we can really love ourselves we can share this sense of touch, which is Spirit in motion, with our lover, and experience a connected unity that brings oneness. It is why making love is so beautifully transcendent.

WORK, EQUALITY, AND PROSPERITY

Our material life has such a big impact on our daily existence that we need to consider how it is affecting our planet, society, and ourselves. We spend so much of our time working hard to put food on the table and clothes on our backs that it is essential we find happiness in what we are doing. But, sadly, this happiness is rare, whether we look at it at an individual or global level. Our current globalized, corporate-dominated, "profit-at-all-costs" economy is certainly not bringing enduring happiness to our world. We need to find a way of living that is nourishing on all levels of our existence, a way that supports our health, wealth, environment, and happiness.

The global view

We live in a world that promises prosperity and we all want a part of it. Not many of us would say, "My life is going really well, I'm broke." We want material wealth to provide for us now and to continue into the future. But our prosperity does not depend just on how much cash we have and cannot be considered in isolation from the rest of the world. It should be seen in the context of how prosperous our neighbors are, how safe and equal our society is, and how healthy our environment.

Over one billion people in the world live on less than $1 per day; average life expectancy in Swaziland is 31, while in Japan it is 82. This sounds neither prosperous nor equal. We know that those societies perceived to be the most equal (such as Japan, Sweden, Norway, and the Netherlands) have better life expectancy, literacy, children's welfare and higher levels of trust than in the less equal societies (such as the UK, Australia, and the USA). These, in turn, have higher rates of murder, teenage pregnancy, obesity, infant mortality, and mental illness.

If my economic community is poor then my social community will also be impoverished and my own personal prosperity suddenly means much less. Prosperity needs to be shared: it is about greater equality, less poverty, less hunger, more social justice, more hopes for peace in the world. It helps us feel more secure that the world is becoming a better place: safer for our children, fairer for our fellow citizens.

But here's the conundrum: if we want greater equality we need the economy to continue growing so that the poorer sections of society can become more prosperous. However, our pursuit of prosperity is based on a false dream of perpetual economic growth, which continues at the expense of the stability of the ecosystem, as well as that of a more equal distribution of wealth. In effect, we are reducing the chances of the good life in the future.

So what can we do and what can business do? Not only do we need to find ways of generating prosperity without harming the environment on a global, business, and individual level, but we, as individuals, also need to find meaning in our life without such a dependence on consumer goods. We must work together to build communities that share in the sense of the common good. Our new religion – individualistic consumerism—is the antithesis of what we require to thrive in the future. For its part, the business community should consider measuring effectiveness on a "triple bottom line": to aim for not just economic profit and general prosperity, but for social and environmental benefit, too. Environmental authors Robert and Christine Prescott-Allen write: "A society is thought to be sustainable when both the human condition and the condition of the ecosystem are satisfactory or improving. The system improves only when both the condition of the ecosystem and the human condition improve." Their words sum up the ethos of this book: look after yourself so that your life improves and look after your world—in the widest sense—so that it improves.

Work fulfillment

Our work life must mirror our society's striving for prosperity. It needs to offer an opportunity for flourishing; the ability to earn enough to pay for our lifestyle, to care for our children, and to give security; the chance of contributing to our community; the potential for creating something better in the future; the freedom to share in the whole while owning the responsibility for our own part. If we can find a job that offers this then we increase the chances of finding fulfillment, which is, after all, what life is all about. I know it's easy to say—but it can be done.

I don't want to sound too idealistic, but as an eternal idealist I can't help it. I like to think of the "magic wand" effect: if you could wave your magic wand, what would you want? What career would fulfill all of the above criteria and help you achieve your dreams? Perhaps you stopped following your dreams because of practical reasons; did life conspire to send you on a different path? Why not dream again and revaluate what you really want to do? By giving yourself choice and being totally clear with what you want you have a much higher chance of finding it. You certainly won't discover it by luck, but you may by planning it out and by being discerning about what is important to you. Clarity can blow away the mist and help you find what you want. And this is what Ayurveda wants for you: for you to be truly fulfilled on a material, emotional, and spiritual level.

LIFE AND DEATH

And so we come to the biggest question of all: how do we feel about our own mortality? To most of us it is an overwhelming and frightening concept, but we all think about it from time to time, even if only to say, "I'll deal with that later." Yet what we believe happens to us after death affects every moment of our lives, a case of "my life is eternal" versus "have one life that is finite." Having an eternal view of life, where the body dies but a part of us lives on, brings a spaciousness and timelessness to everything we do, while thinking that life is finite gives us an urgency that can close the space to the potential of what life can bring us. I am not saying either perspective is right or wrong, but I just want to emphasize how our beliefs about death can fundamentally alter how we live.

Ayurveda embodies the essence of how to live because contained within its belief system is the everyday reality of death. Death is not seen as the "end" of life, but as part of a continuum, a steady stream of consciousness that endures for ever and ever. This is the "silent witness" within all of us that can observe life from a slight distance. It is that private person deep inside who can gaze into the mosaic of our life and observe without reaction as the pattern unfolds. And this means living in the presence of the pain, fear, and reality of death in the same breath as the celebration, joy, and ecstasy of life. Neither side of the coin is more real than the other.

It is possible to develop this more open way of being by nurturing a creative relationship with the nature of pain, suffering, and death. By expanding your awareness of life you will develop constructive attitudes and positive approaches to the opportunities and challenges that come your way so that you are better prepared. However brilliantly you deal with life, it will involve the challenges of pain, ill health, suffering, and death, and so you might as well get to know them.

Simple practices, such as breathwork, meditation, and immersion in nature, can bring this understanding into our everyday lives, so that from each experience we have the possibility to integrate and grow. Engaging in life fully, even when it is raining grief, takes us ever deeper into the eternal source of love that resides within us. For anyone wanting to explore how we can integrate our sufferings within the heart of love more deeply, I recommend the writings of Stephen and Ondrea Levine (see Selected Bibliography, p.248).

Along with change, death is one thing that we can guarantee will happen in our lives. Yet the fear and taboo surrounding it can mean we become paralysed by the idea of it. Most of us are subconsciously gripped by a fear of death, which is natural. However, by embracing this fear we can liberate ourselves from this burden and actually feel more alive. A classic yogic meditation involves sitting in a graveyard contemplating our own inevitable death. (Its extreme even involves meditating on a corpse.) This may sound shocking to our fragile sensibilities, but if we can come to understand the transient nature of this physical body and our limited existence within it we can gain insights into the true nature of our being. When we recognize our mortality we can deeply appreciate being alive and respect every precious moment.

We can become open to the wisdom that we are not the body, nor the mind, but eternal spirit, pure and beautiful. Having a greater proximity and deeper relationship to the potential of our own death also means we can live more fully in the present, cherishing each moment for the uniqueness that it embodies. We can savor each experience afresh: a drop of dew, the smell of a freshly flowering rose, the kiss of a lover. Through knowing death we can hold a beacon of love for every moment that has just passed, for every friend who has lost a friend, for every child who has lost a parent, for every parent who has lost a child; for any suffering anywhere. Death teaches us the true meaning of life ... and that is love.

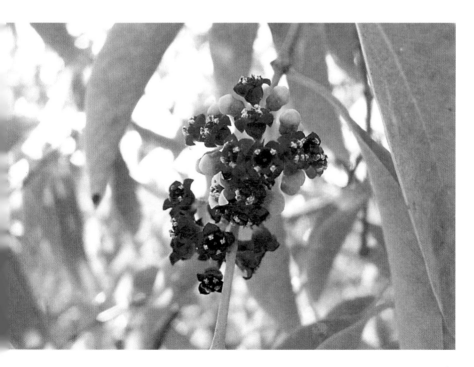

Dancing Shiva

The Hindu deity Shiva takes many forms. As Nataraja, or "Lord of the Dance," he plays out the creation, preservation, and dissolution of the universe. Every moment new experiences arise. Shiva Nataraja reminds us that everything which comes into creation must also pass out of it. He shows us that life can be hard and that the only way through is to find a space of inner stillness among the ebbs and flows around us.

Dancing in a ring of fire, Shiva Nataraja is "held" within the arms of the universe. The beat of the drum sounds life, while the glowing fire destroys it. Yet benevolence is always near. His central hand is kept open, a blessing that offers protection from ignorance and suffering. Shiva proves his ability to offer such protection, as only a master of his own self can, by dancing on the demon of his own suffering. And all this while balanced on one leg: pure stillness, perfect balance. Thoughts and feelings come and go. He is present to it all, but grasps at nothing. As the eternal energy of the universe he manifests, evolves, and absorbs all that has come before it. And it carries on.

The cobra twirling around his neck holds the power of all nature within itself. It is the life force, pure energy, pure *shakti*. Having harnessed this potency, Lord Shiva is in control of nature. Engaging her, caressing her, he unleashes nature's mighty force, all the time maintaining a look of someone who is in charge of their destiny: blissful, peaceful, easy.

This is you, too, dancing through your every day, beating out the tune of your life and singing your song, the one held within your history, your story: family, friends, lovers, children, land, sky, and sun. Hopes and fears tenderly stand on your old patterns and habits, for they are your past and you are born anew every moment. They are burned and transformed as you live in stillness. It's always empty in there. It's always connected in there. And in this space you find your heart. And in this space you find yourself.

You are the dance.

BRINGING IT ALL TOGETHER

As we draw to a close I offer you the soul of Ayurveda. It contains all of the insights that anyone could ever need for a fulfilling life, all wrapped up in its exquisite simplicity: follow your heart, let your witnessing wisdom arise, and study the nature of nature. Remember to organize your life so that it is easier to follow some of Ayurveda's guidance: surround yourself with life-giving foods, nurturing friends, and creative space for yourself to flourish. Learn about your constitution and start to experiment with your diet, habits, and lifestyle so that you can really know how Ayurveda's theories apply to you in your life. Follow your intuition with regards to what suits you when you eat, drink, sleep, and love. Use visualization and meditation techniques to instill inner peace of mind. Use the constitutional diet and relaxation practices to help you find your true path.

For this is what Ayurveda is all about: following your inner nature, in balance with your outer world, so that your spirit can blossom. It's important to bear in mind that Ayurveda sets a pretty high standard, which is not always easy, or even possible, to reach. But by instilling your intention at the core of your being there is no doubt that you will find everything that you seek.

Are you looking for me?
I am in the next seat.
My shoulder is against yours.
You will not find me in the stupas, not in Indian shrine rooms,
nor in synagogues, nor in cathedrals:
not in masses, nor kirtans, not in legs winding around your own neck,
nor in eating nothing but vegetables.
When you really look for me, you will see me instantly –
you will find me in the tiniest house of time.

Kabir says: Student, tell me, what is God?
He is the breath inside the breath.
KABIR, FIFTEENTH-CENTURY INDIAN MYSTIC POET

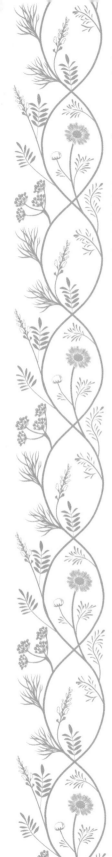

PUKKA PRACTICE

AWARENESS OF THE PRESENT

Being able to stand back from your life for a moment provides a wonderful perspective: most things don't seem quite as worrying or stressful when viewed from a distance. Meditation helps you develop this ability to "stand back" and instills a very powerful guide within you. This is your "witness," your ability to watch your life, yet be involved with your life, but without being totally embroiled in it.

The practice of inner silence

Swami Satyananda Saraswati teaches this six-part meditation as a means of developing deep inner stillness. Its effectiveness comes from its ability to guide you through the phases of meditation, from sense withdrawal to concentration, to meditation and beyond. It is an active meditation that quickly leads to inner peace and is extremely helpful for analyzing and releasing destructive thought and behavioral patterns. Like all meditations, it is best learned with a teacher. You can also use a CD (*see* Resources, p.251) or record this text yourself and play it back.

Make sure you are sitting comfortably: rooted below, still above. Close your eyes. Do a brief body-scan and soften any tension: feet-legs-hips-back-spine-shoulders-neck-back of head-top of head-forehead-eyelids-ears-nose-mouth-whole face-throat-chest-belly. Notice your breath and let it flow in and out.

Exploring your senses

The first part of the practice involves awareness of the founding elements of the universe as well as your immediate world. It takes you on a journey from the start of universal evolution to your present awareness and on to your natural state of inner peace.

Become aware of the outside world. Be mindful of your senses: sound, touch, sight, taste and smell. Let them intermingle and caress your perception. Feel the world around you.

Now move your awareness to your ears. Sound travels through the subtlest element of space, Ether; it is expansive, subtle, light, infinite. Notice the sensation

Hear the flow of sounds around you. Don't actively listen; let the vibrations come to you. You don't need to recognize the sound, just make note of it. Notice sounds coming from different directions, from far away and nearby. Be aware of the pitch and volume: subtle sounds, the invisible sounds. Completely tune in to hearing sound. Hear the silence.

Move to an awareness of feeling, which is carried by the element of Wind. Wind is light, mobile, and fluctuating, a little denser than Ether. The sensation of touch travels through the skin and nerves like the breeze rippling the surface of the water. Observe any sensations you become aware of: the pressure of your body on the ground; your clothes touching your skin; your eyelids touching, your lips touching, your breath touching your nostrils and expanding your belly. Feel your heart beating. Notice the sensation of feeling throughout your entire body.

Next become aware of sight on the back of your eyelids. Sight is generated by the element of Fire, which is hot, sharp, penetrating, luminous, ascending, and dispersing. Notice any color or images appearing. Let the kaleidoscopic spectrum dance before you. Let the colors beaming out of the fire of life sparkle. Let the shapes swirl. Notice how vast your internal field of vision is.

Then move to an awareness of taste. Your ability to taste comes from the element of Water; it is fluid, heavy, wet, lubricating, cool, cohesive, and subtle. It is denser than Fire. What do you taste in your mouth, at the front and at the back? If you need a little help, generate saliva and swallow, tasting the flavor in your mouth. Is it sweet, bitter, metallic? Is it dry or sticky? What taste are you experiencing?

Finally, bring your awareness to your sense of smell. Your ability to smell is due to the Earth element, with its qualities of thickness, density, solidity, heaviness, and stability. Earthy and dense objects emit aromas. Bring your awareness to your nostrils; observe the different scents carried from the earth to you. Are they sweet or wet, light or heavy? Breathe the earth and become aware of your sense of smell.

Everything you notice is always there, it's just that your awareness is not consciously sensitive to it. Now indulge each of your senses: sound, touch, sight, taste, and smell; ears, skin, eyes, tongue, and nose. Circle your awareness for a few moments until you arrive at your breath.

Journeying inward with your breath

Your breath is the link between your body and your mind. So often unconsciously flowing, it is also within your grasp. Whenever you want to you can connect with your breath and control it.

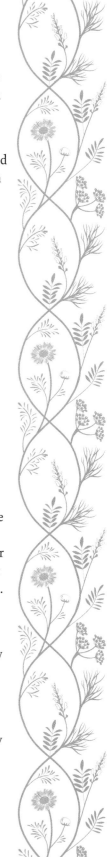

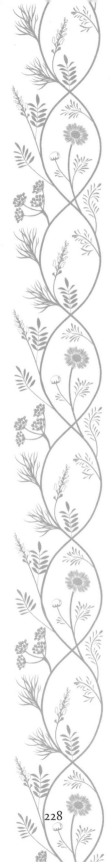

With your awareness on breath draw your senses inward and focus on the space within you. Bring your awareness to your eyebrow-center (*see* Strength and Stillness, p.166) and watch the pattern of your thoughts. Stay here for a few minutes and then move on to the next phase.

Watching the river flow

Your objective self is watching your thoughts in the mirror of your mind. There is a continual stream of thoughts. Now, imagine yourself sitting on a large rock in the middle of a shallow river. As the water flows gently by, begin to watch your thoughts sailing along. You have no agenda and are just watching the play of your mind unfold. Internalize your watching and notice the effects your thoughts have on how you are feeling, where you are feeling, and what you are feeling. How are your thoughts and feelings connected? Just let your thoughts come; don't get involved. Be dispassionate, nonjudgmental; just witness. Let your thoughts   come and let them go. It's all the same. All that letting go … continual letting go … eternal letting go.

Inner peace

Now you can start the practice of holding consciously on to thoughts. Choose a spontaneously arising thought. Let it go. Catch a spontaneously arising feeling. Let it go. Fixate on a spontaneously arising physical sensation. Watch it go. You are aware that, for example, "I am thinking of food" or "I am thinking of love." Keep holding, keep releasing. Keep pulsing your thoughts, feelings, and sensations like this until they are almost imperceptible. Subtle mind. Still mind. Clear mind. Thoughts arising, thoughts dissolving. The sea of thought dissolving in the stream of the mind.

Now move from selecting random thoughts to choosing a subject. Choose something that is challenging you. With your witness firmly awake, think all about this topic: from above, from below, from the side and from within. How does it look? How does it make you feel? How does it make others feel? Why is it such an issue? Can you imagine it being different? What do you need for it to be different? What does it look like when it is different? Can you make it different? When can you do this? When you have thoroughly investigated this subject, let it go. Notice how you feel. Be aware of the calmness and clarity in your heart. The stillness.

Now choose another thought. Choose something that is inspiring you. With your witness firmly awake, think about this idea from every angle: from the past, the present, and the future. How does this inspire you? What can you learn from this experience? What qualities does it have? Can you see these qualities in other areas of your life? Can you infuse your life with these qualities? How can you do this? When can you infuse your life with these qualities? Now let these ideas go. Feel the stillness.

Innerness
Now just be with yourself. Experience what you feel. Wholeness, integration, interconnection. Just what is. You. Stillness. Bliss.

The great return
From this state of deep inner silence, begin to externalize your awareness. Notice how you are feeling. Notice any sounds you can hear, any feelings you can feel. Come back to your body. Come back to the room you are in. Feel yourself in it. Take some deep breaths. Connect your whole body and breathe. Start to make some small movements. Roll your shoulders. Now rub your hands together until your palms are hot and place the palms of your hands over your eyes. Feel the warmth. And behind your hands slowly open your eyes. You are back in your room.

Take the awareness you have at this present moment out into your life. Carry your witness within you. Carry the silence within you.

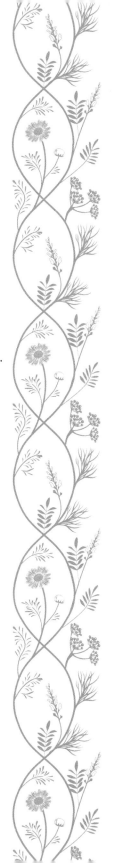

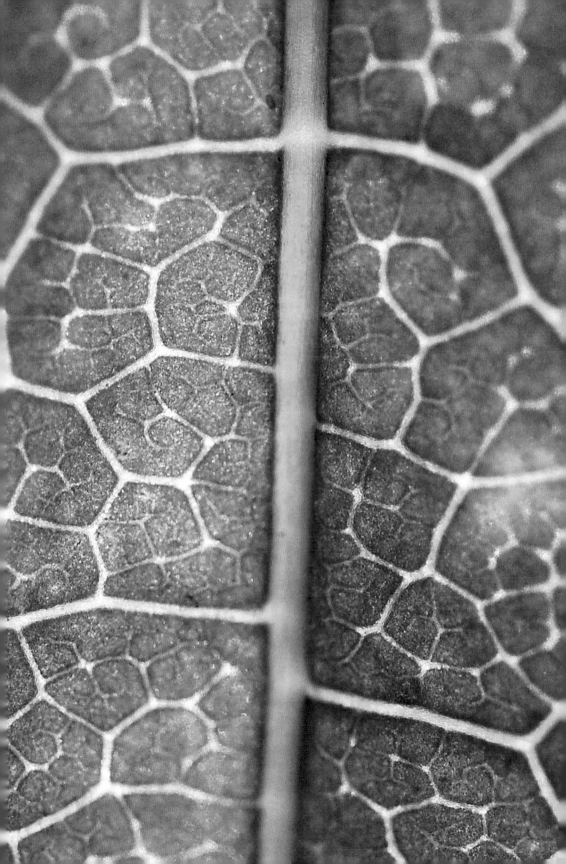

THE PUKKA PANTRY

- ❀ Grains
- ❀ Beans
- ❀ Vegetables
- ❀ Fruits
- ❀ Nuts and seeds
- ❀ Meat and fish
- ❀ Oils
- ❀ Herbs and spices
- ❀ Sweeteners
- ❀ Other common foodstuffs
- ❀ Superfoods
- ❀ Specialist "pukka" herbs

Grains

Amaranth Sweet and bitter in taste, cooling and light to digest. Amaranth reduces all three *dosha*s and is beneficial for the lungs and digestive tract. It has a higher content of easily assimilated calcium than milk and is a great tonic food for *vata* types.

Barley Sweet to taste and cooling and drying in energy. Barley reduces *pitta* and *kapha* but can increase *vata* unless used in watery soups. It has a "lightening" effect on the body and acts as an effective diuretic. Barley water (¼ cup of barley decocted for 30 minutes in 4 cups of water) treats painful urination, clears swellings, reduces edema (swelling), and brings down a fever and inflammations. Barley strengthens digestion and assists the gall bladder and nerves. Unroasted, it increases the bulk of the stools and acts as a mild laxative; when roasted it stops diarrhea. Roasting also makes barley, the most acid grain, more alkaline. It is best to use whole barley, not pearl barley.

Buckwheat Sweet, astringent, and pungent in taste, warming and heavy in quality. Buckwheat increases *vata* and reduces *pitta* and *kapha*. It strengthens digestion but should not be used in *vata* conditions involving spasms, nervousness, dizziness, or emotional imbalance. Buckwheat is high in rutin, which can strengthen capillaries, reduce blood pressure, and stop bleeding. Roasting makes it more alkaline (and more delicious).

Corn Sweet to taste and warm, dry and light in quality. Corn increases *vata* and *pitta* but reduces *kapha* and is traditionally eaten in winter in India with mustard greens as a warming food. It strengthens the kidneys and boosts sexual infirmity, while also strengthening the heart. It is low in niacin and so should be cooked with foods that help niacin absorption, such as limes, peanuts, and wheat. The blue variety is slightly cooling and considerably more nutritious than the yellow one.

Millet Sweet and salty to taste, cooling, dry, and light in quality. Millet increases *vata* and *pitta* but reduces *kapha*. It is mildly diuretic, helping to clear excess *kapha* fluids, and strengthens digestion.

Oats Sweet to taste, and warming, moist, and heavy in quality. Oats can help to reduce *vata* and *pitta* but their moistness can increase *kapha* and extinguish the digestive fire in those with low *agni*. A superb restorative for the nervous system, they also nourish the reproductive system and tonify immunity for weak and deficient people. Their ability to nourish the deeper tissues helps to heal the bones and connective tissues.

Oats can help to reduce cholesterol and strengthen the heart and are also a great demulcent wash for dry and itchy skin.

Quinoa Sweet, bitter, and astringent to taste, cooling, light and soft in quality. Quinoa reduces all three *dosha*s and is one of the best healing foods. It nourishes the deeper reproductive tissues and benefits the digestive tract. It has the highest protein content of any grain and has more calcium than milk.

Rice (basmati) Sweet to taste, aromatic, cooling, and light in quality. Basmati rice reduces all three *dosha*s. It is the best grain for healing the digestive tract, and especially good for clearing heavy stagnation due to high *kapha*.

Rice (brown) Sweet to taste, heating and heavy in quality. Brown rice can reduce *vata* but increases *pitta* and *kapha*. However, *vata* types should not eat too much, as it can be hard to digest. Rice cakes are drying and aggravating to *vata* but reduce *pitta* and *kapha*.

Rice (wild) Wild rice is sweet to taste, warming and harder than other types of rise to digest. While it is very nutritious and suits all three constitutions, wild rice must be very well cooked for *vata* types.

Rye Bitter and astringent to taste, with heating, dry, and heavy qualities. Rye can aggravate *vata* and *pitta* but reduces *kapha*. A very nourishing grain, although hard to digest, it benefits the liver and clears stagnation.

Wheat Sweet in taste, cooling, heavy, and moist in quality. Wheat reduces *vata* and *pitta* but strongly increases *kapha*. It is very nourishing and energizing, particularly tonifying the reproductive tissue. It can be calming to the heart and nervous system, helping with anxiety and high *vata*, but must be avoided by those with excess fluids, weight, and growths. A common source of intolerance, this is largely due to the stale and rancid quality of most wheat flour and the method of modern baking with yeast rather than natural leaven and sourdough. Ensure that you use a freshly ground supply of flour or try spelt, which is more warming and easier to digest.

Beans

Aduki beans Sweet, sour, and astringent to taste, aduki beans have a mildly warming effect and are heavy and drying. They increase *vata* but reduce *pitta* and *kapha*. They are an excellent tonic for the kidneys and for clearing watery stagnations from the body.

Chickpeas Sweet and astringent to taste, with cooling, dry, and heavy qualities. Chickpeas increase *vata* but reduce *pitta* and *kapha*. A good source of iron, they nourish the blood and strengthen the heart.

Kidney beans Astringent and sweet in flavor, warming and heavy in quality. Kidney beans increase *vata* but reduce *pitta* and *kapha*.

Lentils (red) Astringent and sweet to taste, cooling and light in quality. Red lentils increase *vata* but reduce *pitta* and *kapha*. A mild diuretic, they also nourish the heart and assist with blood circulation.

Mung beans Sweet and astringent to taste, cooling, light, and dry in quality. Mung beans reduce *vata* and *pitta* but can increase *kapha* in excess (although are fine in small amounts). The easiest to digest are the dehulled "yellow split" mung. An excellent detoxifying food for all the *dosha*s, it cleans the tissues, strengthens the eyes, tonifies the heart, drains dampness, and clears toxic heat from the body.

Soybeans Sweet and astringent to taste, cooling and heavy in quality. Soybeans increase *vata* and *kapha* but can reduce *pitta*. Tofu is made from fermented soybeans. It is sweet and astringent to taste and is very cold, heavy, and wet in quality. It can be tolerated by *vata* and *kapha* if well marinated and well cooked. It reduces *pitta* and its extreme coldness can be used to bring down a fever when used as a poultice. Tempeh is made from fermented soybeans, and is astringent and warming, so it increases *vata* and reduces *pitta* and *kapha*. Soy milk is sweet, astringent in taste, and heavy and dry in quality. It strongly aggravates *vata*, obstructing the flow of *vata* downward, and increases *kapha*. Soy sauce is fermented and slightly sour and astringent. Its salty nature reduces *vata*, but increases *pitta* and *kapha*.

Tempeh *see* Soybeans

Tofu *see* Soybeans

Vegetables

Alliums (onions, garlic, radishes, leeks) Pungent, sweet, heating, heavy, nourishing, and tonifying when cooked, alliums reduce *vata* and *kapha* and increase *pitta*. Raw onions and garlic strongly aggravate *vata* and *pitta* but reduce *kapha*. As good sources of sulfur and inulin, they are particularly beneficial for helping the balance of flora in the digestive system.

Artichoke (Globe) Astringent, sweet, and heating, globe artichokes lead to an increase in *vata* and a reduction in *pitta* and *kapha*.

Artichoke (Jerusalem) Astringent, sweet, bitter, cooling, dry, light, and rough, Jerusalem artichokes increase *vata* and reduce *pitta* and *kapha*. They are notoriously hard to digest, especially the skins.

Asparagus *see* Superfoods

Avocado Astringent, cooling, heavy, soft and oily, avocado reduces *vata* and *pitta* and increases *kapha*.

Beet *see* Roots

Brassicas and leafy green vegetables (such as broccoli, Brussels sprouts, cabbage, celery, cauliflower, chard, Good King Henry, kale, mustard greens, lettuce) Bitter, astringent, cooling, light, and dry, tending to increase *vata* and reduce *pitta* and *kapha*. Spinach, when cooked, is astringent, sour, heating, heavy to digest, diuretic, and laxative, reducing *vata* and *kapha* but aggravating *pitta*. When eaten raw in salads, leafy greens aggravate *vata* and *kapha* but can be balancing to *pitta*.

Carrot *see* Roots

Corn Astringent, sweet, heating, light, and rough, corn aggravates *vata* and *pitta* and reduces *kapha*.

Cucumber Sweet, cooling, and light, reducing *vata* and *pitta* and increasing *kapha*.

Eggplant *see Solanaceae*

Fennel bulb Sweet, sour, cooling, light, diuretic, and laxative, reducing all three *dosha*s.

Green beans Sweet and astringent, light to digest, and slightly cooling, green beans balance all three *dosha*s.

Ladies' fingers Sweet, astringent, cooling, and mucilaginous (slimy), okra (also known as ladies' fingers) can reduce all three *dosha*s.

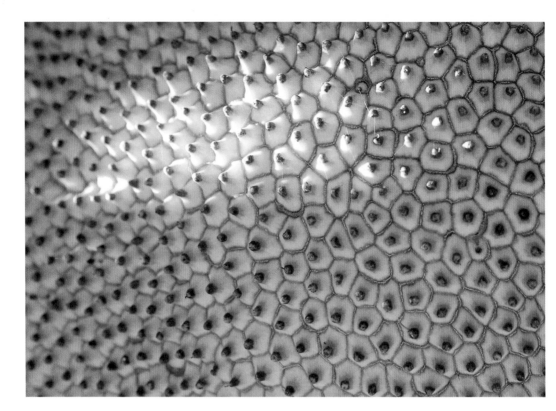

Mushrooms Astringent, sweet, cooling and heavy, increasing *vata* and reducing *pitta* and *kapha*.

Olives Sweet, sour, heavy, and warming, olives can reduce *vata* and increase *pitta* and *kapha*.

Peas (fresh) Sweet, astringent, cooling yet hard and slow to digest, peas can increase *vata* and reduce *pitta* and *kapha*.

Parsnip *see* Roots

Peppers *see Solanaceae*

Potato *see Solanaceae*

Pumpkin *see* Squash and pumpkin

Roots (beet, carrot, parsnip, rutabaga, sweet potato, turnip) Sweet, warming, heavy, grounding, moistening, and nourishing, root vegetables generally reduce *vata* and increase *pitta* and *kapha*. When eaten raw, they can aggravate *vata* as they are hard, cold. and difficult to digest.

Rutabaga *see* Roots

Seaweeds Salty, sweet, cooling, heavy, mucilaginous (slimy), nourishing, and detoxifying, seaweeds reduce all three *dosha*s. They contain fourteen times more calcium and 200 times more iron than any land vegetable. They reduce hard masses in the body, cleanse the lymph, benefit the thyroid, heal the mucous membranes, and assist with weight loss. Eat at least 1g per day.

Solanaceae **(eggplant, chile, peppers, potato, tomato)** Eggplants are astringent, bitter, heating, heavy to digest, increasing *vata* and *pitta* and reducing *kapha*. Peppers are sweet and astringent, heating and dry which can aggravate *vata* but reduce *pitta* and *kapha*. Pepper skins can be very indigestible and aggravate *pitta*. Potatoes are sweet, astringent, dry, light, and very hard to digest, aggravating *vata* and reducing *pitta* and *kapha*— *vata* types should cook with warming spices and ghee to offset these qualities. Tomatoes are sour, sweet, heating, hard to digest, and aggravate all three *dosha*s. Chiles are hot, heating, sharp, and can aggravate all three *dosha*s in excess, though a little is fine for *vata* and *kapha*.

Squash and pumpkin: Sweet, warming, heavy, grounding, and strengthening, all varieties of squash and pumpkin reduce *vata* and *pitta* and increase *kapha*

Sweet potato *see* Roots

Tomato *see Solanaceae*

Turnip *see* Roots

Watercress Pungent, bitter, sweet, heating, watercress reduces *vata* and *kapha* and increases *pitta*.

Zucchini Astringent, sweet, cooling and moistening, reducing *vata* and *pitta* and increasing *kapha*.

Fruits

Apple Astringent, sweet, sour, cooling, light, and rough, apple aggravates *vata* but reduces *pitta* and *kapha*. Baking an apple with raisins, cinnamon, and brown sugar can strengthen the lungs and reduce *vata*.

Banana Sweet, heavy, soft, mucus-forming, banana reduces *vata* and increases *pitta* and *kapha*.

Berries (blackberries, black currants, blueberries, cranberries) Mainly sour, heating, and light, berries reduce *vata* and increase *pitta* and *kapha*. If sweet they reduce both *vata* and *pitta* and increase *kapha*. *See also* Superfoods.

Cherries Sweet, astringent, sour, heating and light, cherries are of benefit to *vata* and *kapha* but they can aggravate *pitta*.

Coconut Sweet, cooling, and demulcent, coconut reduces *vata* and *pitta* and increases *kapha*. Coconut milk is a superb tonic for *vata* and *pitta*, helping to rebuild after deficiency and increase reproductive fluids. *See also* Oils.

Cranberries *see* Berries

Dates Sweet, cooling, heavy, nourishing, and aphrodisiac, dates reduce *vata* and *pitta* and increase *kapha*.

Fig Sweet, cooling, heavy, nourishing, and aphrodisiac, reducing *vata* and *pitta* and increasing *kapha*. Figs are extremely healing to the digestive tract and are useful in treating dry constipation and intestinal inflammation.

Grapes Sweet, sour, astringent, cooling, moistening, strengthening, and aphrodisiac. Grapes reduce *vata* and *pitta* and increase *kapha*. They cleanse the blood and clear heat from the system.

Grapefruit Sour, heating, and acidic, grapefruit increases *pitta* and *kapha* but can benefit *vata*.

Lemon Sour, heating, and digestive, lemon reduces *vata*, mildly increases *pitta*, and significantly increases *kapha*. Do not use if *pitta* is aggravated.

Lime Sour, cooling, and moistening, lime reduces *vata* and *pitta* and increases *kapha*.

Mango Sweet, heating, and nourishing, reducing all three *dosha*s when eaten in moderation but aggravating *pitta* and *kapha* when consumed in excess. Mango is both a laxative and a diuretic and clears heat from the body.

Melon Sweet, cooling, and heavy, melon can benefit *vata* and *pitta* and, because of its hydrophilic (water-loving) quality, it can aggravate *kapha*.

Orange Sweet when ripe, sour when underripe, heating, heavy, and difficult to digest, orange reduces all three *dosha*s when eaten in moderation, and aggravates *pitta* and *kapha* when consumed in excess.

Papaya Sweet, sour, heating, and heavy, papaya reduces *vata* and increases *pitta* and *kapha*.

Peach Sweet, sour, astringent, heating, heavy, and moistening, peach reduces *vata* and increases *pitta* and *kapha*.

Pear Sweet, astringent, cooling, and drying, pear increases *vata* and reduces *pitta* and *kapha*. Cooking offsets these qualities for *vata* types.

Pineapple Sweet, sour, heating, and heavy, pineapple reduces *vata* and increases *pitta* and *kapha*.

Plum Sweet, sour, astringent, heating, and heavy, plum reduces *vata* but aggravate *pitta* and *kapha*.

Pomegranate Sweet, sour, astringent, and cooling and reduces all three *dosha*s. Pomegranate has a specific affinity for the blood tissue. *See also* Superfoods.

Prunes Sweet, cooling, mucilaginous (slimy), and laxative, prunes reduce to all three *dosha*s.

Raspberries Sweet, sour, astringent, and cooling, raspberries increase *vata* and (in moderation) can calm *pitta* and aggravate *kapha*.

Rhubarb Sour, heating, heavy, and laxative, rhubarb reduces *vata* and increases *pitta* and *kapha*.

Strawberries Sour, sweet, and astringent, heating and heavy, strawberries can aggravate all three *dosha*s when consumed in excess.

Watermelon Sweet, cooling, and heavy, watermelon increases *vata* and *kapha* and reduces *pitta*.

Nuts and seeds

Cashew, hazelnut, macadamia, pecan, pine, pistachio, walnut Sweet to taste, heating, heavy, and oily in quality. These nuts are building, strengthening, and aphrodisiac tonics that boost fertility. They reduce *vata* and increase *pitta* and *kapha*. As they are hard to digest they can aggravate *vata* when consumed in excess. High in oils, they can easily become rancid and should be dry roasted before eating. For almond *see* Superfoods.

Flaxseed Sweet, demulcent, and heavy. A superb laxative, flaxseed reduces *vata* and *pitta* and increases *kapha*. Its heavy and wet qualities can extinguish the digestive fire (*agni*) if used in excess and this can aggravate *vata*.

Peanut Sweet, heating, hard, and oily. Very hard to digest, peanuts slow digestion and can impair the liver. While beneficial for the lungs and for lubricating the intestines, they are grown with heavy inputs of chemical fertilizers. Susceptible to heavy processing, rancidity, and aflatoxin infection, peanuts are the lowest-quality nut and should only be eaten in small amounts from organic sources.

Pumpkin seed Sweet and bitter to taste, heavy and hard in quality, pumpkin seed is excellent for clearing worms and nourishing the reproductive system.

Sesame seed Sweet, bitter, and astringent to taste, heating, heavy, and oily in quality. The black variety is a superb blood tonic and a gentle demulcent laxative. Its heating properties can aggravate the blood in individuals susceptible to skin problems.

Sunflower seed Sweet and astringent in taste, cooling and oily in quality, sunflower seed reduces all three *dosha*s.

Meat and fish

Beef Heavy and heating, beef reduces *vata* and increases *pitta* and *kapha*.

Chicken Sweet, heating, and light, white chicken meat reduces *pitta* and *kapha* and increases *vata*, while the dark meat reduces *vata* and increases *pitta* and *kapha*.

Fish Saltwater fish is sweet, salty, heating, and reduces *vata* while increasing *pitta* and *kapha*. Crustaceans especially aggravate *vata* and *pitta* in excess. Freshwater fish is sweet, astringent, and heating and can balance all three *dosha*s but should only be had in moderation by *pitta* and *kapha*.

Lamb Heating and heavy, lamb increases all three *dosha*s.

Pheasant Sweet, rich, heating, and heavy to digest, pheasant aggravates all three *dosha*s.

Pork Heating and heavy, pork increases all three *dosha*s.

Turkey Sweet, astringent, cooling, and light, white turkey meat reduces *pitta* and *kapha* and increases *vata*, while the dark meat reduces *vata* and increases *pitta* and *kapha*.

Dairy

Butter Sweet and sour to taste, heating and oily in quality, butter reduces *vata* and *pitta* and increases *kapha*. It is considered to be nourishing and building, although it increases constipation.

Buttermilk Sweet, sour, and astringent to taste, heavy and demulcent in quality, buttermilk reduces *vata* and *pitta* and increases *kapha*. Ayurveda recommends that it should be drunk after meals as a digestive for aiding assimilation and easing piles. Buttermilk is best if obtained from churning yogurt as a by-product from making butter. If you cannot get this, dilute one part yogurt to two parts water. Adding salt, cumin, or cilantro transforms this into an elixir of health.

Cheese Sour to taste and heating and heavy in quality, cheese reduces *vata* and increases *pitta* and *kapha*. Soft cheese aggravates *pitta* less, while hard cheese increases constipation. Cottage cheese is lighter, less heating, and easier to digest.

Eggs Sweet, heating, and heavy to digest, eggs reduce *vata* and increase *pitta* and *kapha*. The yolk is more warming and strengthening than the white.

Ghee (clarified butter) Cooling and sweet, oily and heavy, ghee (clarified butter) kindles the digestive fire (*agni*) and balances all three *dosha*s, but should not be used in *kapha* conditions with clear, white discharges and or when there is general congestion. It contains a balance of easy-to-digest, short-chain fatty acids that are essential for healthy skin, nerves, and cells. Specifically, it lubricates and moistens the tissues, clears toxins, and is an all-around rejuvenative. Ghee is ideal for healthy cooking due to its high "smoke point," which means it does not produce damaging free radicals and, when eaten as part of a vegetarian diet, it can help raise "happy" HDL cholesterol and reduce "lousy" LDL.

Milk Sweet to taste, cooling, heavy, unctuous and congesting, milk reduces *vata* and *pitta* and increases *kapha*. Though it is hard to digest, it is considered a superior food in Ayurveda as it is the refined juice of plant essence. It can greatly benefit the convalescing patient, children, and deficient individuals. It directly nourishes *ojas* and builds reproductive strength. However, do not consume milk cold from the refrigerator or with other foods, especially fish, sour foods, salt, and leafy green vegetables. Pasteurized, homogenized and nonorganic milk creates toxins, so take from organic

sources. Goat milk is lighter to digest than cows milk, benefits the lungs and strengthens the whole body. Like all dairy, it can still create mucus.

Sour cream Sour, heating, heavy, and unctuous, sour cream benefits *vata* and can increase *pitta* and *kapha*.

Yogurt Sweet and sour to taste, warming, wet, and heavy, yogurt reduces *vata* and increases *pitta* and *kapha*. It benefits digestion, nourishes fertility, and cures diarrhea. However it is a tricky food to digest properly as it is very fickle. According to Ayurveda, it should never be eaten at night, in the winter, or very hot summer, cold from the refrigerator or without mixing it with ghee, honey, sugar, mung beans, or amla fruit. This is because it has a unique negative property that obstructs the flow of the water element in the body and blocks the channels of circulation. This hydrophilic (water-loving) quality leads to mucus buildup, water stagnation, and congestion. Store-bought yogurt is often very sour and this excessively aggravates *pitta* and *kapha*. Eat only small quantities: 2–4 tablespoons at a time.

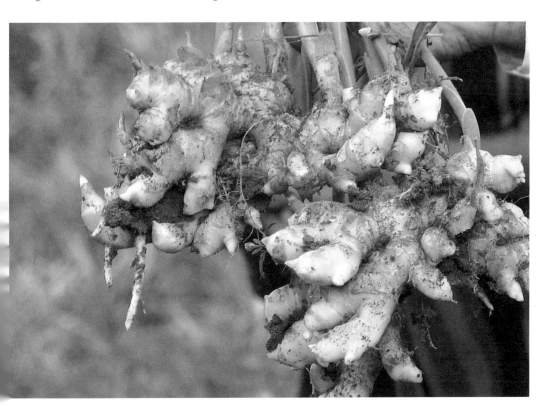

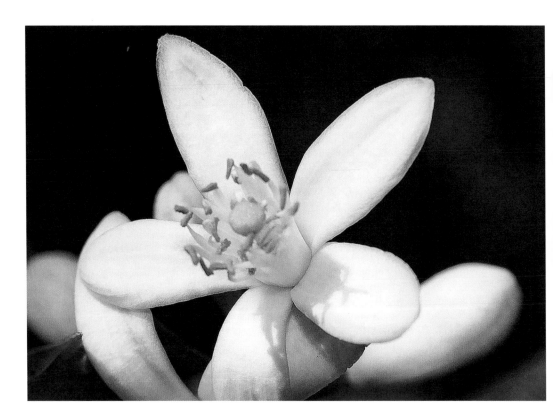

Oils

Coconut Sweet, cooling, heavy, and unctuous, coconut oil reduces *vata* and *pitta* and increases *kapha*. It contains lauric acid, the fatty acid nearest to mother's milk in structure, and is very high in the medium-chain fatty acids that increase metabolism and help balance weight. It is a superb oil for use in cooking.

Corn Sweet, astringent, heating, and heavy, corn oil aggravates *vata* and *pitta* and can reduce *kapha* as it is slightly drying.

Flax Sweet, astringent, heating, and slightly drying, flax oil benefits all three *dosha*s. It is very high in omega-3 essential fatty acids, and it must never be used for cooking.

Ghee *see* Dairy

Hemp Sweet, cooling, heavy, and unctuous, hemp oil balances all three *dosha*s. The seed of this infamous plant is a superb demulcent laxative. The oil also has a perfect balance of omega-3, -6, and -9 essential fatty acids, and is high in gamma linolenic acid (GLA) and stearidonic acid,

pointing to its use as an anti-inflammatory, nervous restorative, and cardiac tonic.

Olive Sweet, cooling, and heavy, olive oil reduces *vata* and *pitta* and increases *kapha*. It can cause cellulite when used in excess.

Sesame Sweet, bitter, and astringent to taste, sesame oil is warming and lubricating in quality. It is Ayurveda's favorite oil for reducing *vata*; it increases *pitta* and mildly increases *kapha*. It is a superb tonic for the digestive fire (*agni*), skin, and hair. Sesame oil also nourishes the mind and improves the intellect.

Sunflower Sweet and astringent, cooling, light, and soft, sunflower oil reduces all three *dosha*s.

Herbs and spices

Anise Pungent, heating, and light, anise reduces *vata* and *kapha* and increases *pitta*. It is especially good for the digestion and lungs.

Asafetida Also known as "devil's dung" due to its omnipervasive sulfurous smell. Pungent, heating, drying and sharp, asafetida reduces *vata* and *kapha* and increases *pitta*. It is very effective for stopping digestive, menstrual, and nervous pain.

Black pepper Pungent, heating, drying, and sharp, black pepper reduces *vata* and *kapha* and increases *pitta*. It is especially good for the digestion and lungs.

Cardamom Pungent and sweet, with light, and drying qualities that balance all three *dosha*s, cardamom always tastes best when the pod is lightly crushed. The seeds contained inside are great to chew throughout the day to help your digestion and keep your mind awake. Use it as antidote to the cloying quality of dairy products and sweet foods.

Celery seed Pungent, heating, light and sharp, celery seed reduces *vata* and *kapha* and increases *pitta*. It is especially good for the digestion and is a very effective tonic for the nervous system.

Chili (cayenne) Pungent, hot and drying, chili powder (cayenne) reduces *vata* (when used in moderation) and *kapha* and increases *pitta*. It is very useful for warming circulation, increasing expectoration and enhancing absorption of nutrients (when used in small quantities).

Cinnamon Spicy and sweet with a heating and drying quality that balances all three *dosha* (but can aggravate *pitta* in excess). Cinnamon is a superb spice to invigorate circulation and warm digestion. Recent research has validated its age-old use for reducing blood-sugar levels and resisting weight gain. It is a true tonic that protects and gives strength.

Clove Pungent, heating, light, and oily, clove reduces *vata* and *kapha* and increases *pitta*. It is very effective for removing fungal and bacterial infections from the digestive system as well as opening the channels of the heart (in an Ayurvedic sense).

Coriander Pungent, sweet, and slightly bitter, coriander balances all three *dosha*s. The leaves are more cooling and the seeds more warming. Coriander is a wonderful remedy for helping to clear irritating heat toxins from the body. A cool tea of the seeds can be great for urinary irritation and cystitis, and the leaves are used to help reduce allergies and clear toxins.

Cumin Known as *jiraka* in Sanskrit, meaning "digestive spice," this slightly warming, aromatic, and pungent spice balances all three *dosha*s and helps to stop intestinal spasms, remove toxins, and awaken your mind.

Dill Bitter, astringent, heating, and light, dill balances all three *dosha*s and is a very useful light seasoning to kindle the digestive fire and clear mucus accumulation.

Fennel This sweet seed is warming, balancing all three *dosha*s and helping to build digestive strength. Having hundreds of tiny flowers, the aroma of fennel lightens digestion and, like its ascendant flower head, it spreads and moves outward, thus preventing congestion and stagnation in the abdomen and chest. The tea is an ideal way to benefit from fennel, useful for helping children's digestive colic and encouraging the flow of a new mother's breast milk.

Fenugreek Pungent, bitter, and heating, fenugreek reduces *vata* and *kapha* and increases *pitta*. It is very good for encouraging digestion and regulating cholesterol levels (in larger amounts of more than 1¼ ounces).

Garlic *see* Vegetables, *Alliums*

Ginger Spicy, sweet, warming, and light, ginger reduces *vata* and *kapha* and can increase *pitta*. When using ginger, think "digestion, lungs and circulation." Its digestive benefits are legendary: it warms and strengthens the digestive system, and increases digestive fire (*agni*) and the secretion of digestive enzymes. It is useful for keeping the digestive system clean by preventing nausea (morning, postoperative, and travel sickness), flatulence, griping pains, and sluggish digestion. Fresh ginger especially benefits a cold exterior (such as when you feel cold), while dry ginger warms the inner body, clearing toxins, and improving "cold" mucus aggravations.

Mint Sweet, cooling, and light, mint balances all three *dosha*s. The aromatic leaf is a famous digestive that stops spasms and eases digestive discomfort. Mix into summer soups for a delicious lift. It is a good example of how helping your stomach can help your mind, as they are both responsible for "digesting" our experiences. A cup of mint tea instantly strengthens digestion and clears your mind.

Mustard seed Pungent, heating, light and oily, mustard seed reduces *vata* and *kapha* and increases *pitta*. As well as benefiting digestion, the seed helps to clear mucus from the lungs.

Saffron Sweet, astringent, bitter, heating, dry, and light, saffron reduces all three *dosha*s. It is the most expensive spice, but potentially the healthiest. Its red color points to its benefit for the blood. Saffron has a long tradition of treating heart problems, relieving menstrual pain. and lifting your mood. Its high water-soluble carotenoids levels give it a potent antioxidant capacity.

Turmeric The spice of spices. Traditionally used in Ayurveda for over 2,000 years to heal the joints, frozen shoulder, digestion, liver, heart, brain, skin impurities, and wounds, this golden yellow root is full of the potent flavonoid curcumin and other yellow pigments that act as cellular protectives and systemic rejuvenatives. High in flavonoids and with over 100 clinical studies attesting to its ability to protect and nourish the body, turmeric has gained the reputation of one of nature's most potent remedies for many age-related degenerative diseases such as cancer, diabetes, Alzheimer's, arthritis, and asthma. Its ability to clear the blood of toxins benefits anyone exposed to high amounts of pollutants and stress. Use it in your cooking every day or, because its main components are fat soluble, add it to warm almond milk for a delicious golden drink.

Sweeteners

Barley malt Sweet, cooling, and unctuous, barley malt reduces *vata* and *pitta* but its unctuous and sticky nature increases *kapha*.

Honey Heating in quality, honey reduces *vata* and *kapha* and increases *pitta*. It has a special scraping ability that clears toxins and excess fats from the tissues.

Jaggery A mineral-rich form of condensed cane sugar, jaggery is heating and strengthening. It aggravates *pitta* and *kapha* and reduces *vata*.

Maple syrup Sweet, cooling, and light, maple syrup reduces *vata* and *pitta* and increases *kapha*.

Molasses Energetically similar to jaggery, molasses is also an excellent blood tonic. It reduces *vata* and increases *pitta* and *kapha*.

Refined white sugar The cooling quality of refined white sugar reduces *pitta* and aggravates *vata* and *kapha*. When used in excess it creates undigested toxins (*ama*), and so should be avoided.

Other common foodstuffs

Chocolate Sweet, bitter, astringent, warming, congesting, and heavy, chocolate increases all three *dosha*s when mixed with milk and sugar. Used as pure cocoa powder it is a medicine that calms the nervous system and strengthens *ojas*.

Coffee Bitter, astringent, heating, and penetrating, coffee aggravates *vata* and *pitta* but its stimulating properties can help reduce *kapha*.

Salt Salty, sweet, heating (apart from saindava rock salt, which is cooling), heavy, wet, and penetrating, salt reduces *vata* and increases *pitta* and *kapha*. Its heavy and grounding qualities help *vata* move downward. Salt is an appetite stimulant, toxin remover, channel opener, laxative, emetic, and it clears mucus. In excess it causes water retention and can irritate digestion. It is also contraindicated in skin diseases, acidity, and high blood pressure caused by water retention.

Tea Bitter, astringent, light, and drying, tea increases *vata* and *pitta* and reduces *kapha*. Black tea is fermented and more stimulating, while green tea is steamed and cleansing.

Yeast Sour in taste, warming and light in quality, the concentrated nature of yeast aggravates all three *dosha*s and should therefore be avoided by everyone. It promotes bloating and weakens digestion, promoting the proliferation of candida (thrush). Use natural leavenings and sourdoughs instead.

Superfoods

The designation "superfood" is given to foods that are exceptionally nutrient-rich. Taken in combination, they give enhanced healing effects.

Almond Sweet to taste, heating, heavy, and oily in quality, almonds are the most superior nut, benefiting the lungs, skin, digestive tract, and fertility. Their concentrated mineral content also makes almonds very nourishing for the bones, nails, and hair. Soaking overnight and removing their *pitta*-irritating skin makes them into a cooling, enzyme-rich superfood that boosts *ojas*. Peel and eat or blend with some water, rice milk, saffron, and honey for a rejuvenating tonic drink.

Aloe vera juice Sweet, bitter, cooling, and juicy, aloe vera balances all three *dosha*s. It has an amazing mixture of more than 200 constituents, including phytonutrient polysaccharides, enzymes, glycoproteins, eighteen amino acids, twelve vitamins, and twenty minerals. Polysaccharides have been shown to benefit immunity, reduce inflammation, improve cellular metabolism, and lubricate the intestines. Aloe vera is the most wonderful intestinal healer, useful in treating acidity, ulcers, and Irritable Bowel Syndrome. Traditionally, aloe vera is one of Ayurveda's most renowned fertility rejuvenators, known as "the princess" in India. It is also a fantastic skin tonic that nourishes, soothes and heals. It is considered to have a special ability to transport nutrients deep into every tissue and so is often used as a "carrier" for other remedies.

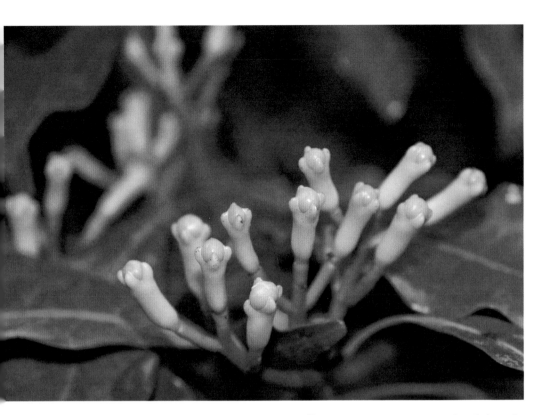

Asparagus Balancing to all three *dosha*s, asparagus is considered to be one of Ayurveda's healthiest vegetables. Its soothing, demulcent, and juicy nature lubricates all the membranes in the body, removing *vata* dryness; its bitter and sweet taste is cooling and removes *pitta* heat; and its diuretic properties clear any *kapha* dampness and water retention.

Berries Berries, such as blackberries, blueberries, bilberries, elderberries, and acerola and goji berries, are mainly sour, heating, and light, reducing *vata* and increasing *pitta* and *kapha*. They are packed with vitamins, phytonutrients, and phenolic compounds such as anthocyanins (pigments which give the fruits their characteristic red, blue, and purple vibrancy). Berries have renowned antiaging and antioxidant benefits, as they help to protect our cells. They do this in many ways: by facilitating the absorption of harmful oxidative products; protecting the precious lipids in the cell membrane; slowing the reproduction of rogue cells; and immobilizing mutated cells. Their juices stop the blood forming clots by reducing platelet levels, giving circulatory system support and benefits to those at risk from strokes and heart attacks. They also reduce inflammation and strengthen the body's collagen tissue.

Broccoli sprouts Bitter, astringent, cooling, light, and dry, broccoli sprouts tend to increase *vata* and reduce *pitta* and *kapha*. These "super-sprouts" are associated with the health of the bowel, breasts, bladder, ovaries, lungs, and liver. Sprouts are a good source of glucosinolates, which are converted by friendly bacteria in the digestive system into healing isothiocyanates. These in turn activate the "Phase 2" enzymes in the liver that help to process and neutralize harmful oxidizing and carcinogenic substances. One such glucosinolate, sulforophane, has been shown to modulate and influence cancer-related genes. Freshly grown and freeze-dried sprouts have more than 10mg per gram of glucosinolates and 4,500μg per gram of sulforophane. Just 3½ ounces of broccoli sprout powder gives you the equivalent sulforophane of an entire 100g serving of fresh broccoli.

Chlorella Sweet, bitter, cooling, light and dry, chlorella reduces *pitta* and *kapha* but can aggravate *vata* in excess (more than ¼ ounce per day). It is a hugely beneficial alga, which evolved out of the "cosmic soup" approximately 540 million years ago. It has a tough outer wall that has to be "cracked" to release its potent nutritional essence. This strong cell wall reflects its ability to strengthen our own "outer wall" or immunity, a theory that is validated by its ability to stimulate the immune-boosting protein, interferon. Its incredible ability to absorb solar energy gives it an impressive nutritional profile: an especially high chlorophyll content (three percent), 2.5 percent Chlorella Growth Factor (a unique compound known to support the immune system), 58 percent protein, all the B vitamins, high levels of essential nutrients such as Vitamins A and D, folic acid, iron, iodine, magnesium, and zinc, and concentrated doses of omega-3, -6, and GLA. The abundance of nucleic acids makes it invaluable for cellular growth, repair, and renewal. Others amongst its array of health benefits include cleansing the liver, protecting the heart, replenishing the nervous system, building energy, nourishing blood, reducing inflammation, and enhancing regeneration.

Flower pollen Having a complex spectrum of tastes, including sweet, sour, astringent, salty, and bitter, flower pollen is a building and nutritious food that can help to balance all three *doshas*. This wonderful substance has all the known nutrients necessary for human survival. It is gathered by bees from the stamens of flowers and collected from hives as small pellets. These contain approximately 35 percent vegetable protein, around eighteen vitamins, 25 minerals, 60 trace elements, and all amino acids, and are also full of enzymes, co-enzymes, plant growth hormones, essential fatty acids, and slow-releasing carbohydrates. Pollen is extremely rich in vitamins B (including B12), C, D, and E, and in lecithin, cysteine, and golden yellow carotenes, which are metabolic precursors of Vitamin A. Many of the nutrients in flower pollen have been scientifically documented for their ability to strengthen immunity, reduce aging, rejuvenate the nerves, brain, and heart, and counteract the effects of radiation and chemical toxins.

Spirulina Sweet, bitter, cooling, light, and dry, spirulina reduces *pitta* and *kapha* and increases *vata* in excess (more than ¼ ounce per day).This microscopic freshwater blue-green plant (actually, it's a photosynthesizing "cyanobacteria") has a unique profile that nourishes, supports, and gently strengthens the body. It is one of the most nutritionally dense foods in the world, containing over 100 nutrients, including the antioxidant phycocyanin and an easily digestible spectrum of vitamins, minerals, amino acids, proteins, antioxidants, essential fatty acids, and nucleic acids. Its high protein content (60 percent) includes all the amino acids and means that, gram for gram, it has 300 per cent more protein than animal meat, and has 80 percent digestibility (beef protein has 20 percent). It is the second-highest source of GLA after mother's breast milk (¼ ounce spirulina provides more than 90mg of the recommended 150–300mg GLA per day), making it useful in heart disease, blood clotting, asthma, arthritis, dermatitis, allergies, diabetes, and nerve repair. Spirulina contains 58 times more iron than spinach, 25 times more beta-carotene than carrots, 300 percent more calcium than milk, and 35 times more phytonutrients than blueberries, and 60 times more than spinach. Phycocyanin, the blue-green pigment responsible for photosynthesis, is a powerful antioxidant that can scavenge free radicals and has also been shown to inhibit cancer-colony formation.

Wheatgrass juice Sweet, bitter, cooling, and light, wheatgrass juice balances all three *doshas* (but can increase *vata* in excess). It is a true gift from nature, containing healthy amounts of bioactive enzymes (which help us digest food and detoxify), superoxide dismutase (an important antioxidant), beta-carotene, lutein, vitamins (A, B12, E, K), and minerals (iron, magnesium, calcium). It also contains high quantities of chlorophyll and mucopolysaccharides that help immunity, build tissue strength, and reduce inflammation. Good for rejuvenating and detoxifying the whole body, it is specifically helpful for blood-building, constipation, intestinal conditions, liver imbalances (including cancer), joint inflammations, obesity, blood-sugar disorders, menstrual irregularities, and fatigued muscles. As cereal grasses are very cooling, anyone who is energetically "cold," such as *vata* or *kapha* types, should take them with caution—chlorella and spirulina may be better suited to their constitutional needs.

Specialist "pukka" herbs

In Sanskrit, "pukka" means "ripe" or, more colloquially, "first-class," "best quality," or "top-notch" and I love these herbs for the gift they bring in helping us to live at our most "ripe"—that is, nearer to our potential.

Amla (*Emblica officinalis*) Sweet, sour, bitter, astringent, and cooling, this broad-spectrum healer is also known as Indian Gooseberry. Amla rejuvenates all three *doshas* and is best used when there is overall weakness in the system. Amla's hallmark as a great healer is its therapeutic flexibility: it is an immune stimulant (beneficial for short-term infections) and also an adaptogen that deeply nourishes immunity to offer long-term protection from degenerative diseases. Its powerful antioxidant capacity can help delay aging and prolong life and is useful whenever there is chronic inflammation and/or weakness in the digestive system, liver, blood, or heart. It is a part of the famous triphala formula (*see* p.245) and also one of the main ingredients in chywanaprash (*see* opposite), which are other good ways to get your dose of amla.

Andrographis (*Andrographis paniculata*) The bitter and drying properties of andrographis reduce *pitta* and *kapha*, helping to lessen inflammation in the liver and to increase bile secretion—in this respect, andrographis has been proven to be more powerful than the more widely known milk thistle. It has also been shown to have beneficial effects for the detoxifying pathways in the liver, helping to protect the activity of antioxidants as well the overall level of glutathione. In addition, andrographis has a positive effect on the immune system, boosting white blood cell production as well as acting against viruses. It is my herb of choice as an acute remedy for colds and flu, helping to clear sore throats, fevers, and upper respiratory tract infections.

Ashwagandha (*Withania somnifera*) Sweet, astringent, warming, and strengthening, Ashwagandha reduces *vata* and *kapha* and can mildly increase *pitta*. Its reputation for promoting inner calm and core vitality makes this the perfect herb for addressing today's lifestyle demands. Ashwagandha is particularly good for those who are anxious and have difficulty sleeping. Its ability to strengthen the blood, build iron levels, keep muscles firm, and increase bone density make it indispensable for slowing aging. This herb also has an incredibly diverse effect on the key stress and hormonal triggers in the body, with an affinity for the adrenal, endocrine, and nervous systems. It has a long history of use in treating immune disorders, hormonal imbalances, thyroid problems, blood-sugar levels, chronic inflammation, and infertility.

Arjuna (*Terminalia arjuna*) Despite being very astringent, arjuna balances all three *dosha*s. One of Ayurveda's "wonder herbs" for strengthening the cardiac muscle, reducing arterial congestion, and lowering blood pressure, arjuna works a bit like the better-known hawthorn berry in that it is similarly used to treat angina, myocarditis, and other heart conditions. Its wound- and trauma-healing properties are renowned for helping the emotional aspect of heart disease and healing "broken hearts" caused by grief.

Boswellia (*Boswellia serrata*) Bitter, astringent, sweet, pungent, warming, and moving, boswellia balances all three *dosha*s. Also known as Indian frankincense, this resin has strong analgesic properties and is used to reduce pain and inflammation—it has a special "scraping" property that removes adhesions and deposits from joints and the channels. It is employed generally when there is inflammation in the joints, lungs, digestive system, and skin and more specifically to treat autoimmune diseases, such as rheumatoid arthritis, osteoarthritis, ulcerative colitis, Crohn's disease, and psoriasis.

Brahmi (*Bacopa monnieri*) Bitter, sweet, and cooling, brahmi balances all three *dosha*s. Named after Brahman, the Universal Consciousness, this herb is renowned for influencing the quality of thought. Clinical studies have shown that brahmi can help increase cognition, memory, and concentration, while also greatly improving anxiety. It is useful when someone is "stuck" in a repetitive cycle of destructive habits, be these dietary, social, or emotional. This is because brahmi brings clarity, which is why it is also used in treating Alzheimer's, ADHD, and autism, or any form of mental illness. Its cleansing properties extend to its specific ability to dredge aluminum and cadmium from the brain.

Chamomile (*Matricaria recutita*) Bitter, sweet, and cooling, chamomile reduces all three *dosha*s. These exquisite yellow flowers are full of the sweetness that can help to relax the nervous system. Chamomile is used as a delicious tea to induce good sleep, settle restless legs, and stop spasms. It also has a mild bitter flavor that makes it a wonderful digestive, helping to ease bloating, cramps, and inflammation throughout the digestive system. Not to be confused with Roman Chamomile (*Anthemis nobilis*), which is much more bitter.

Chywanaprash Sweet, sour, and spicy, nutritious chywanaprash nourishes all three *dosha*s, but can increase *kapha* if taken in excess and *pitta* if it is a particularly hot variety. This delicious and unusual tasting jam has the amla fruit as its main ingredient and is mixed with around 35 other herbs, including ashwagandha, shatavari, the roots of ten trees, cardamom, cloves, cinnamon, and triphala. Chywanaprash is now used to help with all facets of rejuvenation: recovery from disease, improving mental clarity, improving fertility, prolonging life, and delaying aging. It is specifically used for weight loss, breathing difficulties, immune weakness, seasonal infections, and heart disorders. It is high in antioxidants, with one serving of chywanaprash providing 35 percent of daily antioxidant requirements.

Ginseng (*Panax ginseng*) Sweet, sour, and heating, ginseng reduces *vata* and *kapha* and can increase *pitta*. Although it is not specific to Ayurveda, ginseng is one of the ultimate rejuvenating herbs and is an excellent adaptogen. The best stock comes from plants that are at least five years old. The herb is heating and stimulating and should only be used with an appropriately nourishing diet. It raises energy, strengthens digestion, nourishes the heart, improves memory, tonifies immunity, strengthens breathing, improves fertility, and reduces high blood-sugar and cholesterol levels. It should not be used if there are heat signs, such as thirst, headaches, and fevers.

Gotu kola (*Hydrocotyle asiatica*) Bitter, astringent, sweet, and light, gotu kola is balancing to all three *dosha*s. This herb is also known as *mandukaparni*, "the frog-foot-like plant," on account of the webbed foot shape of its leaf and the fact that it loves the water. The shape of the leaf resembles a cross-section of the brain and it does, rather remarkably, improve mental faculties. This creeping plant is used extensively to sooth the redness, swelling, and itching of inflammatory skin diseases. A powerful circulatory stimulant that penetrates deeply into the tissues, it is an effective herb to include in treatment for joint and muscular conditions associated with heat and pain. It has a positive effect on the mind, especially useful when there is an emotional component to the cause of any inflammation: it reduces the stress of trauma caused by a wound, shock, skin disease, or mental fog. As it balances all three *dosha*s, it also removes the "shock" of any *dosha* imbalance. By normalizing the cellular function, it enhances cellular communication and promotes cellular intelligence; I use it in treating Alzheimer's and epilepsy. It is also used to help prevent deep-vein thrombosis.

Licorice (*Glycyrrhiza glabra*) Sweet, bitter, and unctuous, licorice reduces *vata* and *pitta* but can increase *kapha* if too much is used. It is one of nature's most delicious herbs. It is about 50 times sweeter than sugar without affecting blood-sugar swings and is used in traditional medicine as a "harmonizer" to help bring balance to the flavor and effect of a herbal tea. It is slightly cooling and so can help with inflammation in the lungs, digestive system and urinary system. It has a mild demulcent or soft quality that helps to sooth irritation (such as that caused by ulcers) and is renowned for helping to ease mucus congestion and lung inflammation. It is also a strong tonic, helping to nourish the adrenals and can help with exhaustion and strengthening a burnt-out nervous system. Its calming effects on the mind can be easily felt when it is drunk as a tea (0.5–2g per cup); its sweet, soothing and grounding effects are immediately apparent. While there are some concerns about the use of licorice aggravating high blood pressure, this has only been documented with high consumption of licorice sweets or when taking more than 12g per day of the powdered root.

Neem (*Azadirachta indica*) Bitter, cooling, light and dry, neem is one of Ayurveda's best herbs for removing heat and reducing inflammation. Along with its anti-bacterial/-protoazoal/-fungal properties, its cooling energy reduces redness, swelling and pain caused by excess hot *pitta* and wet *kapha*. It therefore has a strong affinity for liver inflammation and skin diseases, especially with redness, suppuration and itching. It is also

beneficial when there is intestinal inflammation caused by parasites or candida imbalance. The seed oil is very useful for fungal infections of the nails when applied every day for three months.

Pippali (*Piper longum*) Ayurveda's favorite warming spice, pippali balances *vata* and *kapha* and increases *pitta*. Also known as long pepper, pippali is one of the three ingredients in trikatu. On its own, its penetrating pungency stimulates the immune system and rejuvenates the digestion and lungs, helping to clear *kapha* congestion and toxins. Its antiamoebic and -giardial properties make it especially beneficial for the gut. The alkaloidal piperine content, along with its essential oils, play a vital role in pippali's ability to help absorb nutrients, digest herbal formulas, and clear mucus from the lungs.

Reishi (*Ganoderma lucidum*) Sweet, bitter, astringent, reishi balances all three *dosha*s. Its potent immune-boosting polysaccharides have earned it the title of "mushroom of immortality." Reishi is used to protect immunity in cancer and chemotherapy patients, but it benefits the lungs, heart, and pancreas, too. This herb is also known as "spirit mushroom," attesting to its ability to strengthen the heart and calm the nervous system, making it a useful aid to sleep and to calm an overactive mind. Reishi also helps more generally to reduce inflammation and cholesterol.

Shatavari (*Asparagus racemosus*) Sweet, bitter, and unctuous, this herb reduces *vata* and *pitta* and can increase *kapha*. Shatavari, literally meaning "a hundred (roots) below," is a perennial plant that has a mass of succulent tuberous roots. Because it is so effective for women's health it has become known as "the woman who has 100 husbands," although it also benefits men's fertility and heals digestion, too. Shatavari is a good example of why it is the person that is treated, not the disease. All reproductive markers improve: it brings strength, is an aphrodisiac, promotes menstruation, improves fertility, reduces miscarriage, nourishes *ojas*, and increases breast milk. Its ability to cool *pitta* makes it helpful where there is excessive bleeding from the uterus, digestive system, or lungs. It is often helpful in the end stages of treatment for endometriosis and polycystic ovary syndrome. Its cooling and moistening properties and its ability to regulate hormone levels make it a perfect herb for treating menopausal symptoms.

Trikatu Pungent and hot, trikatu reduces *vata* and *kapha* and can increase *pitta*. Made from equal parts of dry ginger, black pepper, and pippali, this warming formula awakens digestion, digests, and destroys toxins,

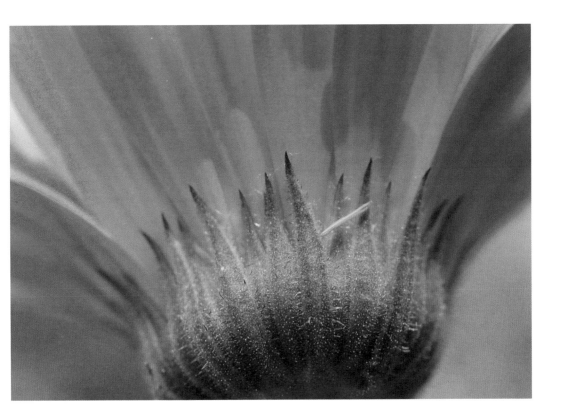

removes fat and obesity, and is an overall rejuvenative, especially to *kapha* and the lungs. Trikatu benefits breathing, alleviates coughs, and asthma, and can be a helpful remedy for hay fever and acute allergic rhinitis as an immediate way of drying up the copious nasal secretions; it also has antiallergenic effects. As it has an affinity for all the orifices of the head, it is used to treat sinus congestion, chronic nasal blockage, a muzzy head, blocked ears, and a sore throat.

Triphala Sweet, astringent, cooling, and balancing to all three *dosha*s, triphala is Ayurveda's most famous formula, made from equal parts of three fruits: haritaki (*Terminalia chebula*), bibhitaki (*Terminalia belerica*), and amla (*Emblica officinalis*). It helps to detoxify and to nourish and is traditionally used to maintain a healthy digestive tract. As a toxin digester it helps to clear a "furry" tongue and fermenting bowel; as an appetizer it brings a healthy desire for food; as a blood cleanser it removes skin blemishes; and as a mild laxative it banishes constipation without causing dependency. It redirects the flow of energy downward, helping your motions and digestion to be regular and is an overall rejuvenative, considered to prolong life. Just 2g of triphala has potent antioxidant activity higher than a whole cup of cherries.

Tulsi (*Ocimum sanctum*) Pungent, bitter, warming, and ascendant, tulsi balances all three *dosha*s (but can increase *pitta* in excess). This leafy member of the mint family is a potent rejuvenating plant that builds immunity, with the ability to lift the spirits, ease depression, and help sleep. Its dispersing action makes it very useful for protecting from seasonal colds and fevers, as it reduces damp *kapha* and cold *vata*. By modulating the inflammation induced by the COX-2 enzyme, it works like other anti-inflammatory drugs—but without the damaging side effects. It is also very useful for tension headaches, allergic irritation, nervous digestion, and the physical ache associated with 'flu and colds.

Vacha (*Acorus calamus*) Pungent, acrid, hot, and penetrating, vacha reduces *vata* and *kapha* and increases *pitta*. This water-loving root has traditionally been used in small quantities for its psychoactive properties. Its acrid and pungent qualities restore the mental faculties of perception and self-expression, removing dullness, depression, and vegetative states. Its ability to open the channels in the mind is invaluable for the treatment of addictions. *Vacha* means "speech" in Sanskrit, and small doses of it help clear mental fogginess. It is best used under the guidance of a practitioner.

GLOSSARY

Acute Any disease with a sudden onset, intense symptoms, and brief duration.

Agni The digestive fire, with the function of regulating digestion, absorption, and assimilation.

Allopathy The system of medicine that uses treatments that oppose the pathology of a disease (e.g., anti-inflammatories to treat inflammation); also refers to modern orthodox medicine in general.

Alterative A herb that alters the chemical state of the blood; blood-cleanser.

Ama Undigested food or experiences that create disease-forming toxins.

Anabolic The building phase of metabolism, associated with **kapha**.

Analgesic Pain-reliever.

Antibiotic Opposes life and kills pathogenic bacteria.

Antispasmodic Relieves muscular spasms and contraction.

Aromatic A fragrant herb that contains essential oils, which tonify digestion and reduce flatulence.

Ashtanga Hridaya Samhita Or Ashtanga's Heart of Medicine, *The Eight-Limbed Heart Sutra* written by Vagbhatta c.600 a collated work on the essence of Ayurveda.

Atharva Veda The last of the four *Vedas*, ancient Indian religious texts.

Atman Your individual self, as opposed to **brahman**.

Ayurveda The traditional medical system of India, meaning the "science of life."

Basti Autoenemas; one of the six cleanses (*see* **shatkarma**).

Bhagavad Gita Sacred Hindu scripture, describing the nature of reality in a conversation between Lord Krishna and Arjuna.

Bhavaprakasha Written by Bhavamishra in 1596 CE— the most important Ayurvedic *materia medica* treatise, listing the energetics of herbs and foods.

Brahma nadi The channel that carries **kundalini** (divine energy) to the crown **chakra**.

Brahman Your universal self, as opposed to **atman**.

Buddhi Intellect.

Carminative A herb that relieves gas, spasms, and helps digestion.

Catabolic The destructive phase of metabolism, associated with **pitta**.

Chakra An energy center linking the physical and subtle body. Also related to the plexuses, from where nerve fibers spread throughout the body.

Chandogya Upanishad A primary philosophical text of the Hindu religion.

Charaka Samhita Or *Charaka's Compendium*: the first Ayurvedic text to be recorded in writing in the second century BCE, supposedly edited by the Ayurvedic doctor, Charaka. It is considered to be a compendium of all previous Ayurvedic thought.

Chidakasha The space of consciousness, behind the eyebrow-center or "third eye" **chakra**.

Chronic A disease with gradual onset, long-term symptoms and gradual changes.

Demulcent A soft and muciligenous herb that protects the mucous membranes.

Dhammapada A collection of verses gathered from the words of Buddha that beautifully express his teaching.

Dhanvantri The Lord of Ayurveda.

Dhauti Internal cleansing; one of the six cleanses (*see* **shatkarma**).

Dosha Constitutional type, of which there are three: **vata**, **pitta**, and **kapha**. When balanced they are responsible for good health, but when imbalanced they act as "faults" and can cause illness.

Guna The ten pairs of opposing attributes that Ayurveda uses to describe the different qualities of matter. *See also* **trigunas**.

Hatha Yoga Pradipika Twelfth-century early yoga text describing various yoga practices.

Hridaya The heart; also the seat of feelings, sensations, the soul, mental operations, and divine knowledge.

Kapalabhati A brain-cleansing breathing practice; one of the six cleanses (*see* **shatkarma**)

Kapha One of the three **doshas**, with qualities of Earth and Water. It is heavy, wet, and cold, lives in the stomach, and is responsible for nourishing the mucous membranes, bones, joints, heart, and memory.

Karma The universal principle of cause and effect.

Kundalini Cosmic manifestation of divine energy that is said to flow up channels around the spine.

Laxative A herb that causes a mild bowel motion.

Manas Part of the mind that conceptualises and analyses; includes memory.

Markandeya Purana Hindu religious text styled as a discussion between two sages, Markandeya and Jaimini; includes the itinerant musings of Lord Dattatreya.

Materia medica Literally, "the materials of medicine"— the study of the drugs or substances that are used to treat disease. Commonly used to refer to books that document the properties of herbs.

Mitochondria The structures responsible for energy production in cells.

Moksa Spiritual emancipation, self-realization.

Nauli Abdominal massage; one of the six cleanses (*see* **shatkarma**)

Nervine A herb that has an affinity for nourishing and calming the nervous system.

Neti Nasal cleansing; one of the six cleanses

(see *shatkarma*).

Ojas "Vital essence," or the quality that maintains the inherent immunity and strength of the body.

Panch karma The five traditional cleansing techniques of therapeutic emesis, purgation, enemas, nasal cleansing, and bloodletting.

Panchmahabhuta The five great elements of Ether, Air, Fire, Water, and Earth that make up the material world.

Patanjali's Yoga Sutras A third-century text to describe the eight "limbs" of yoga.

Pathology The typical behavior of a disease.

Pitta One of the three *doshas*, comprising Water and Fire. It is hot, wet, and light and its main site is the small intestines. It is responsible for the metabolic processes of the body. When healthy it adds zest, clarity, and energy to life but when aggravated it creates burning, inflammation, and anger.

Prakriti The individual constitution and inherent nature of every person; as opposed to *vikriti*.

Pramahamsa Yogananda Founder of the Self-Realization Fellowship, author of *An Autobiography of a Yogi* and a revered saint.

Prana The "breath of life," or life force, absorbed from the air, food, and nature. It is responsible for vitality and cellular communication.

Pranayama The yogic practice of breathing with awareness. The focus is on extending the length of breath and balancing the rhythm; **yoga**.

Qi The "vital force" in traditional Chinese medicine, bringing warmth and energy to the body.

Qigong The traditional Chinese practice of exercises developed to regulate, build, and move *qi*, the life force.

Ramayana An Indian epic depicting the life of Lord Rama, woven with the cultural themes of duty (*dharma*), love, and the meaning of life.

Rajas The quality of nature responsible for movement, passion, and energy; one of the *trigunas*.

Rasa Literally, "taste"; it can also by translated as "essence," "juice," "sap," "lymphatic fluid," "flavour," and "delicious" and so carries with it all those associations.

Rasayana Rejuvenation (literally, "the path of juice"), a principle objective of Ayurveda.

Rejuvenative A substance used to tonify and nourish the whole system.

Rig Veda An ancient Indian collection of sacred hymns from the Bronze Age, c.1500 BCE.

Samanya-vaisheshika The principle of "like increases like," or "opposites balancing opposites," the cornerstone of Ayurvedic practice.

Samkhya One of the six schools of classical Indian philosophy from which Ayurveda draws its cosmological understanding of matter and evolution.

Samkhya Karika A first-century Indian philosophical text.

Sankalpa Intention or resolve; part of the relaxation practice of Yoga Nidra.

Sattva The quality of nature reflected in compassion, light, and intelligence; one of the trigunas.

Saundaryalahari Eighth-century devotional poem eulogizing the wonder of Lord Shiva's companion, Shakti.

Sedative A substance that tranquilizes the nervous system.

Shakti Meaning "energy"; represents the dynamic feminine vitality throughout the universe; also (as one of the manifestations of Parvati) the natural and balancing opposite to Shiva.

Shatkarma The six cleanses of traditional yoga practice: *basti, dhauti, kapalbhati, nauli, neti, trataka*.

Stimulant Increases metabolism, circulation, and the function of an organ.

Sushruta Samhita A detailed surgical text written around c.100–500 by the great Ayurvedic teacher Sushruta.

Tamas The quality of nature that reflects dullness, inertia, and darkness; one of the trigunas.

Tantra A spiritual path utilizing all of the senses for deifying the body. Successfully practiced, this results in being carried across to the other side of existence, the shores of liberation.

Tejas The essence of the fire element. The result of the perfect digestion of all pitta-natured foods that gives consciousness and clarity to the mind.

Tonify The effect of a food, herb, or exercise that "tones" and strengthens the quality of a tissue, organ or system.

Trataka Steady gazing, a tool for meditation; one of the six cleanses (see *shatkarma*)

Trigunas The three metaphysical universal forces: *sattva, rajas,* and *tamas*; also known as the three mind qualities.

Vasodilator A herb that encourages the relaxation of blood vessels.

Vata One of the three *doshas*, made from the elements of Ether and Air. It is light, dry, and cold and resides principally in the large intestine. It is responsible for all movement in the nervous system, muscles, heart, and mind.

Vikriti The current state of someone's health or the present state of imbalance; as opposed to *prakriti*.

Vrikshayurveda A c.sixteenth-century Ayurvedic text by Surapala, focusing on the care and treatment of plants and trees.

Yoga The practice of unifying the mind and body, self, and cosmic self. Commonly practiced as postures (*asanas*), breathing techniques (*pranayama*), and meditation practices (*dhyanam*) to harmonize the health of the body and mind.

SELECTED BIBLIOGRAPHY

For a complete list of references please look on
my website: www.apukkalife.com

Abramson, J. *Overdosed America: The Broken Promise of
American Medicine*, Harper Perennial, 2005

"Alliance for Natural Health," Sustainable Healthcare
White Paper, 2008

Atreya. *Practical Ayurveda*, USA, Samuel Weiser, 1998

Bensky, D. and Gamble, A. *Chinese Herbal Medicine:
Materia Medica*, USA, Eastland Press, 1986

Bernard, T. *Hatha Yoga*, India, Rider, 1950

Capra, F. *The Web of Life: A New Scientific Understanding of
Living Systems*, Anchor, 1997

Conze, E. *Buddhism: Its Essence and Development*, Oxford
University Press, 1960

Dash, B. and Sharma, R. *Charaka Samhita*, India,
Chowkhamba Press, 1996

Eliade, M. *Yoga: Immortality and Freedom*, USA, Princeton
University Press, 1958

Frawley, D. and Lad, V. *The Yoga of Herbs: An Ayurvedic
Guide to Herbal Medicine*, USA, Lotus Press, 1994

Gladstar, R. *Planting The Future: Saving Our Medicinal
Herbs*, Inner Tradition, 2000

Griggs, B. *Green Pharmacy: The History and Evolution of
Western Herbal Medicine*, Healing Arts Press, 1981

Harvey, G. *We Want Real Food*, Constable, 2006

Hoffman, D. *Medical Herbalism: The Science and Practice of
Herbal Medicine*, Healing Arts Press, 2003

Holford, P. and Burne, J. *Food Is Better Medicine than
Drugs*, Piatkus, 2006

Jackson, T. *Prosperity Without Growth*, Earthscan, 2009

Kowalski, R. *The Only Way Out Is In*, Jon Carpenter, 2001

Lad, V. *Ayurveda: The Science of Self-Healing*, USA, Lotus
Press, 1984

Lad, V. *Textbook of Ayurveda: Fundamental Principles*,
India, The Ayurvedic Press, 2002

Le Fanu, J. *The Rise and Fall of Modern Medicine*,
Abacus, 1999

Levine, S. *A Gradual Awakening: A Guide to Greater
Awareness*, Gateway, 1989

Levine, S. *Guided Meditations, Explorations and Healings*,
Anchor Press, 1991

Levine, S. *Healing Into Life and Death*, Anchor Press, 1987

Levine, S. *Who Dies? An Investigation of Conscious Living
and Conscious Dying*, Gateway, 1986

Levine, S. and Levine, O. *Embracing the Beloved:
Relationship as a Path of Awakening*, Gateway, 1995

Lovelock, J. *A New Look at Life on Earth*, Oxford
University Press, 1979

Meulenbeld, G., *A History of Sanskrit Medical Literature*,
Holland, Egbert Forsten, 2001

Mills, S. and Bone, K. *The Principles and Practice of
Phytotherapy*, Churchill Livingstone, 2000

Murthy, S. *Bhavaprakasha of Bhavamisra*, India,
Krishnadas Academy, 2001

Murthy, S. *Vagbhata's Ashtanga Hridayam*, India,
Krishnadas Academy, 1991–1995

Pitchford, P. *Healing with Whole Foods: Oriental Traditions
and Modern Nutrition*, USA, North Atlantic Books, 1993

Pole, S. *Ayurvedic Medicine: The Principles of Traditional
Practice*, Elsevier, 2006

Radhakrishnan, S and Moore, C. *A Sourcebook of Indian
Philosophy*, USA, Princeton University Press, 1957

Saraswati, N. *Prana, Pranayama, Prana Vidya*, India, Bihar
School of Yoga, 1994

Saraswati, S. *Hatha Yoga Pradipika: Light on Hatha Yoga*,
India, Bihar School of Yoga, 1985

Schlitz, M. and Amorok, T. *Consciousness and Healing:
Integral Approaches to Mind–Body Medicine*, Elsevier,
2005

Spencer, C. *The Heretic's Feast: A History of Vegetarianism*,
Fourth Estate, 1993

Spiegel, D. *Group Therapy for Cancer Patients*, USA,
Basic/Perseus, 2000

Svoboda, R. *Ayurveda: Life, Health and Longevity*, India,
Penguin/Arkana, 1992

Svoboda, R. and Lade, A. *Tao and Dharma*, USA, Lotus
Press, 1995

Tierra, M. *Planetary Herbology*, USA, Lotus Press, 1992

Tillotson, A, *The One Earth Herbal Sourcebook*, USA, Twin
Streams, 2001

Watson, A. "East–West Perspectives on Education,"
presented at the East–West Centre, University of
Hawaii, June 2005

Watts, A. *Psychotherapy East and West*, London, 1971

Wilber, K. *No Boundary: Eastern and Western Approaches to
Personal Growth*, Shambala, 2001

"World Cancer Report," World Health Organization, 2003

Wujastyk, D. *The Roots of Ayurveda: Selections from the
Ayurvedic Classics*, Penguin, 1998

RESOURCES

If you have any queries regarding this book, please contact Sebastian@pukkaherbs.com and I will be happy to answer any questions. Information about my herbal practice is on my website: www.sebastianpole.com

AYURVEDIC AND HERBAL SUPPLIERS

USA

Banyan Botanicals
High-quality Ayurvedic herbs, ethical suppliers of organic herbs, massage and herbal oils, chywanaprash and more. Superb range of Ayurvedic formulas.
www.banyanbotanicals.com

Herb Pharm
Top-quality organic herbal liquid extracts.
www.herb-pharm.com

Herbalist & Alchemist
High-quality herbs and tinctures.
www.herbalist-alchemist.com

Planetary Formulas
Medicinal herbs from Michael Tierra that combine Western, Ayurvedic and traditional Chinese healing systems.
www.planetherbs.com

AUSTRALASIA

Mediherb
Membership website for qualified healthcare professionals.
www.mediherb.com.au

Herbal Creations Limited
www.herbalcreations.co.nz

EUROPE

Austria
Ayurveda Welt
www.ayurvedawelt.at

Czech Republic
Marksman
www.marksman.cz

Denmark
Naturesource
www.naturesource.dk

France
Abiocom
www.abiocom.fr

Germany
Amla International
www.amla.de

All-Bio
www.all-bio.de

Seva-Ayurveda
www.seva-ayurveda.de

Holland
Holisan BV
www.holisanshop.nl

Hungary
Atma Center
www.atmacenter.hu

Italy
Inner Life
www.innerlife.it

Israel
Alternative Pharma Ltd
www.greenmarks.co.il

Greece
Botanica Herbs Remedy Stores
www.botanica.gr

Latvia
Ezoterika
www,ezoterika.lv

Lithuania
Damodara
www.damodara.lt

Norway
Marianne Willumsen
www.pukka.no

Sweden
Biofood
www.biofood.se

Switzerland
TNCO
www.pukka.ch

UK

Pukka Herbs
Pioneers in the organic Ayurvedic field. High-quality herbs, tinctures, capsules, gugguls, oils and essential oils sourced from organic farms and fairly traded.
Tel: 00 44 (0)1179 640944
www.pukkaherbs.com

PRACTITIONERS & HERBAL ORGANIZATIONS

If you are interested in fulfilling your healing journey I strongly recommend that you work with a qualified professional for treatment.

USA
American Herbalists Guild
www.americanherbalistsguild.com

National Ayurvedic Medical Association
www.ayurveda-nama.org

CANADA
The Ontario Herbalists Association
www.herbalists.on.ca

AUSTRALASIA
National Herbalists Association of Australia (NHAA)
www.nhaa.org.au

EUROPE
Academy of Ayurvedic Studies
www.ayurvedicstudies.nl

Algemene Nederlandse Vereniging voor Ayurveda Geneeskunde (ANVAG)
www.anvag.nl

Ayurveda en France
www.ayurveda-france.org

Verband Europäischer Ayurveda-Mediziner und - Therapeuten (VEAT)
www.ayurveda-verband.eu

UK
Ayurvedic Practitioners Association
Tel: 00 44 (0)1273 500492
www.apa.uk.com

Register of Chinese Herbal Medicine
Tel: 00 44 (0)1603 623994
www.rchm.co.uk

The National Institute of Medical Herbalists
Tel: 00 44 (0)1392 426022
www.nimh.org.uk

Unified Register of Herbal Practitioners
Tel: 00 44 (0)7539 28857
www.urhp.org.uk

AYURVEDIC COLLEGES AND RESEARCH CENTERS

High-quality training to deepen your Ayurvedic or herbal knowledge.

USA
American Institute of Vedic Studies
Courses with David Frawley.
www.vedanet.com

California College of Ayurveda
www.ayurvedacollege.com

East West School of Herbology
Correspondence courses with Lesley and Dr. Michael Tierra.
www.planetherbs.com

The Ayurvedic Institute
A variety of programmes led by Dr. Vasant Lad.
www.ayurveda.com

INDIA
International Academy of Ayurved
Runs good short courses on Ayurveda.
www.ayurved-int.com

Gujarat Ayurved University (Jamnagar), Banaras Hindu University (Varanasi) and Mahatilak Vidyalaya at the University of Pune also offer good degrees in Ayurveda.

UK AND EUROPE
Middlesex University, London
Offers a BSc in Complementary Health Sciences (Ayurveda) in association with the College of Ayurveda.
www.mdx.ac.uk

European Institute of Vedic Studies, France
Courses with Vaidya Atreya Smith.
www.atreya.com

Tapovan, France
An "open university," with some courses taught in English.
www.tapovan.com.fr

European Academy of Ayurveda, Germany
Courses with Mr. and Mrs. Rosenberg.
www.ayurveda-akademic.org

Ayurvedic Point, Italy
Courses with Dr. Antonio Morandi.
www.ayurvedicpoint.it

Swiss Ayurvedic Medical Academy
Courses with Dr. Simone Hunziker and Jean-Pierre Bigler.
www.formation-ayurveda.ch

YOGA CENTERS

Yoga Alliance
International yoga organization listing schools and
registered teachers in the U.S. and Canada.

The British Wheel of Yoga
Find a local teacher, teacher training and online shop.
www.bwy.org.uk

The London Satyananda Yoga Centre
Yoga, meditation and chanting in the tradition of the
Bihar School of Yoga. Good yoga CDs, too.
www.syclondon.com

Sivananda Yoga Vedanta Centers
Beginners' courses, talks, teacher training and yoga
retreats.
www.sivananda.org

COUNSELING AND HEALING
ORGANIZATIONS

British Association for Counselling & Psychotherapy
www.bacp.co.uk

Cognitive Behavioural Therapy
www.babcp.com

Constellation Therapy
www.constellationsolutions.co.uk

Emotional Freedom Technique
www.aamet.org

Psychosynthesis
www.psychosynthesis.org

Relate
www.relate.org.uk

United Kingdom Council for Psychotherapy
www.ukcp.org.uk

AYURVEDA SPAS

Ayush Wellness Spa, Hotel de France, St Helier, Jersey
Tel: 00 44 (0)1534 614171
www.ayushspa.com

Essential Ayurveda Retreats, Halton Holegate, Lincs
Tel: 00 44 (0)1754 830559
www.essentialayurveda.co.uk

Maharishi Ayurveda Health Centre, Skelmersdale, Lancs
Tel: 00 44 (0)1695 51008
www.maharishiayurveda.co.uk

Shyamla Ayurveda, Holland Park, London
Tel: 00 44 (0)20 7348 0018
www.shymalaayurveda.com
Tor Spa Retreats, Ickham, Canterbury, Kent
Tel: 00 44 (0)1227 728500
www.torsparetreat.com

USEFUL WEBSITES

www.bigshakti.com
A superb collection of yoga and meditation CDs from
Swami Shankardev and Jayne Stevenson from this site
based in Australia. Also available from
www.pukkaherbs.com in the EU and
www.banyanbotanicals.com in the USA.

www.chenrezigproject.org
Information about infusing life with loving-kindness.

www.herbsforlife.co.uk
Information about Ayurveda and using herbs.

www.rigpa.org
More on Sogyal Rinpoche's Buddhist teachings.

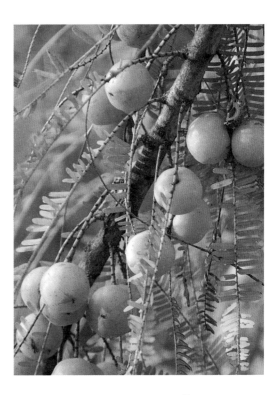

INDEX

acetaldehyde 78
acids 49
adaptogens 121, 128, 129
addictions 144, 146–9
aduki beans 233
aerobic exercise 117
affirmations 141
aflatoxins 80
aging 75, 101
agni (digestive fire) 37, 44–5
  balancing 89
  and immune system 113
  and rejuvenation 131
  and toxins 73
  yoga exercises 127
agriculture 39, 58, 62, 73,
  80, 119
ahimsa (nonviolence) 59
Air 13, 46, 177, 179, 182–3
alcohol 78, 147
aldehydes 78
alkaloids 41
allergies, food 68
alliums 233
almonds 240
aloe vera juice 95, 240
alternate nostril breathing
  162
ama (toxins) 71–3
amaranth 232
amla 122, 242
amphetamines 148
andrographis 93, 121, 243
angina 115
anise 238
anthocyanins 120
antibiotics 56, 104, 106,
  109, 131
antibodies 104
antidepressants 144
antigens 104
antioxidants 40, 56, 57, 60,
  75–6
anxiety 144
apples 235
arjuna 117, 243
artichokes 233
asafetida 238–9
ashwagandha 80, 117, 121,
  122, 168, 243
asparagus 241
aspirin 43
astringent taste 53
atheroma 117
avocados 233
awareness 137, 164, 165,
  214–15, 226–9
bacteria 25, 104
balance: daily constitutional

balancing 89–91
  Gaia Theory 192, 193
  health and ecology 193–4
  homeostasis 25, 76, 103, 151,
    193
  illness as a symbol 212
  pathway of disease 84–5
  strength and stillness 135
bananas 235
barley 232
barley malt 240
basal cell carcinoma 75
beans 54, 233
beef 236
bellows breath 163
Bernard, Claude 25
berries 190, 235, 241
bile 49
bioflavonoids 49
bitter taste 52–3
black pepper 239
blood 95, 185
body massage 170
body–mind 12, 25, 86, 137
  see also mind
boswellia 95, 243
bowels 26, 86
brahmi 95, 168, 243
brain-cleansing breath
  (*kapalabhati*) 88
brassicas 233
bread 41–2
breastfeeding 104
breathing: alternate nostril
  162
  basic breathing practice
    161–2
  bellows breath 163
  brain-cleansing breath 88
  connecting with nature 195
  in corpse pose 127
  humming bee breath 129
  in meditation 164–5, 166–7,
    227–8
  "nostril only" 28
  and rejuvenation 129
  strength and stillness 161–3
  victory breath 162
broccoli sprouts 190, 241
buckwheat 232
Buddha 31, 53, 59, 145, 207,
  209
buddhi (intellect) 137, 138
Buddhism 208–9, 215, 218
butter 236, 237
buttermilk 236

cancer: causes of 118–19
  diet and 113, 118, 120
  free radicals and 75
  herbal remedies 120–1
cannabis 148

cardamom 239
carotenoids 41, 76, 120
the cat pose 155
celery seeds 239
chamomile 168, 243
cheese 236
chemicals, man-made 80–1,
  119
cherries 235
chicken 236
chickpeas 233
chile 234,
chili 239
chlorella 190, 241–2
chlorophyll 185
chocolate 240
cholesterol 115–16, 117
Christianity 145
chywanaprash 122, 129, 130,
  243
cinnamon 239
cleansing 71, 86–99
  Ayurvedic way 86–7
  brain-cleansing breath 88
  cleansing herbs 92–5
  daily constitutional
    balancing 89–91
  Hatha yoga 152, 153
  seasonal detoxification
    and fasting 96–7
  see also toxins
climate 193, 197
cloves 239
cocaine 148
coconut 235
coconut oil 238
coffee 148, 240
cognitive behavior therapy
  141
compassion 207–9
concentration 164
conjugated linoleic acid
  (CLA) 61
consciousness: death and 222
  and the heart 31, 112, 137
  love and 219
  nature and 176
  self-realization 214–15, 217
constipation 26, 141
constitution 11–35
  constitutional health
    questionnaire 32–5
  constitutional tendencies of
    the mind 139
  constitutional types 14–23
  daily constitutional
    balancing 89–91
  discovering 13
  elements 176
    holistic approach 24–5
  and immune system 110
  like increases like 14

opposites balancing
  opposites 14
roots of good health 26–30
taste and 47
yoga for 156–9
consumerism 221
coriander 239
corn 232, 235
corn oil 238
corpse pose 127
cortisol 126, 128
creativity 141
"crimes against wisdom" 83
"cross-linking," free radical
  damage 74–5
cucumber 233
cumin 239

dairy products 55–6, 119,
  236–7
Dalai Lama 207
dancing Shiva 224
dates 235
Dattatreya 160
DDT 80
death 222–3
degenerative disorders 75,
  102
depression 106, 142–4
detoxification 76–7, 82, 86,
  96–7, 185
diabetes 43
diet see food
digestive system 44–5
  balancing 89
  chlorophyll and 185
  cleansing herbs 92
  and immune system 113
  problems 63
  rules for healthy digestion
    38
  stimulation 30
  types of digestion 45
  see also agni (digestive fire)
dill 239
direction, taste and 47
disease: Ayurvedic approach
  to 24–5, 83
  cancer 118–21
  causes of 25, 31, 83
  digestion and 44
  effects of stress 141
  food and 41, 68
  heart disease 114, 115–16,
    144
  illness as a symbol 212
  immune system 104, 110–13
  mind and 140–1
  orthodox medicine 106, 109
  pathway of 84–5
  qualities 13
  rejuvenation and 102

toxins and 72
and Type-B malnutrition 39
and *vata* 15
vegetarian diet and 59–60
DNA 24, 75, 121
doctors 24
doshas 14
constitutional tendencies of
the mind 139
elements 176
pathway of disease 84–5
taste and 47
yoga for 156–9
drugs 25
orthodox medicine 106, 109
painkillers 43
recreational drugs 79, 147–8
safety 109
statins 115–17
toxins 43, 73, 79
treatment of depression
143, 144

Earth (element) 13, 46, 177,
181, 182–3
earth (planet), Gaia Theory
192, 193
eating 29–30
ecology 175–203
connecting with nature
195–6
environmental issues 58, 73,
80–1
Five Great Elements 178–81
Gaia, greed and 192–4
health and 176–7, 193–4
herbal sustainability 186–9
life force (*prana*) and 184–5
natural qualities of the
elements 182–3
seasonal lifestyles 197–203
superfoods 190–1
economics 220–1
ecstasy (MDMA) 148
eggplant 234
eggs 236
elements 13
and constitution 176
"Five Great Elements" 177,
178–83
natural qualities of 182–3
and taste 46
and *vata* 15
elimination 26
emotions: and addiction to
food 149
and depression 143–4
effects of stress 141
heart and 114
illness as a symbol 212
and immune system 105,
112

living from the heart 213
love 218–19
and rejuvenation 128, 131
and toxins 73
endocrine disruptor
chemicals (EDCs) 81, 119
energetics 47
energy: *kundalini* 163
prana (life force) 37, 38,
184–5
environmental issues 58, 73,
80–1
see also ecology
equality 220–1
equilibrium, meditation 164,
165
essential fatty acids 55, 61, 64,
119, 120
essential oils 41, 170
estrogen 119
Ether 13, 46, 177, 178–9,
182–3
exercise 28–9
benefits of 151
nourishing the heart 117
for rejuvenation 126
relaxation routines 154–5
eyebrow-center gazing,
meditation 166
eyes: cleansing 27
and immune system 112
palming 112

fall routine 201–2
fasting 97
fats, in diet 40, 115–16, 119
fennel 233, 239
fenugreek 239
fermented foods 49
fever, qualities 13
fiber, in diet 117, 120
figs 235
Fire 13, 46, 177, 179–80, 182–3
see also agni (digestive fire)
fish 55, 58, 236
"Five Great Elements" 177,
178–83
flavonoids 41, 76
flax oil 238
flaxseeds 236
flower pollen 190–1, 242
food 37–69
addiction to 149
additives 40, 42
antioxidants 75–6
and cancer 113, 118
and detoxification 78, 96
eating 29–30
energetic properties 47
fasting 97
food combining 63
food culture 39–40

healthy relationship with
150
ingredients 54–7, 231–45
intolerances 68–9
kapha diet 67
local food 62
as medicine and as poison
41–3
nourishing the heart 117
organic food 62, 187, 188–9
pitta diet 66
and *prana* (life force) 38,
185
prevention of cancer 120
the Pukka pantry 232–45
qualities 13
and rejuvenation 131, 132–3
roots of good health 29
seasonal, local, and organic
62
superfoods 57, 64, 185,
190–1, 240–2
tastes 46–53
to clear the lungs 79
vata diet 65
vegetarian diet 58–61, 64,
120
what is a food? 41–2
see also digestive system
forces, universal 138
frankincense 121
free radicals 74–7
friends 219
fruits 39–40, 55, 120, 190,
35–6

Gaia Theory 192, 193
Gandhi, Mahatma 59
gardening 196
gazing, meditation 166
genetics 24, 75, 111
germs 25, 104, 113
Gestalt movement 216
getting up 26
ghee 64, 237
ginger 41, 92, 239
ginseng 122, 187, 243
glucose 118
glutathione peroxidase 75
gotu kola 80, 95, 121, 168, 244
grains 54, 58, 64, 119, 232
grapefruit 235
grapes 235
green beans 233
greenhouse gases 58
guggul 80
gum health 26–7
gunas (qualities) 13, 47, 182–3

hallucinogens 148
Hamilton, Alan 186
hangovers 78
happiness 210–11, 213, 214–
17, 220
Hatha yoga 152, 153
healing, mind and 128
health 12
constitutional health
questionnaire 32–5
and ecology 176–7, 193–4
integrated model of
health care 109
roots of good health 26–30
see also disease
heart: Ayurvedic view of 114
and consciousness 31, 112,
137
heart disease 114, 115–16,
144
and immune system 112
living from the heart 213
nourishing 117
heavenly stretch 154
hemp oil 238
herbs 56
adaptogens 121, 128, 129
bitter herbs 52
cleansing herbs 92–5
herbal remedies for cancer
120–1
herbal teas 57, 117, 131
nourishing the heart 117
the Pukka pantry 238–40
pungent herbs 51
rejuvenating herbs 122–5,
129
for relaxation 168–9
sustainability 186–9
to stabilize the mind 80
traditional herbal medicine
(THM) 107–9, 186
vegetarian diet 64
heroin 148
Hinduism 152
Hoffmann, David 193–4
holistic approach 24–5
holons 176
homeostasis 25, 76, 103, 151,
193
honey 57, 240
hormones 12
effects of stress 141
endocrine disruptor
chemicals (EDCs) 81, 119
hormone replacement
therapy (HRT) 79
and immune system 105
humming bee breath 129
hunger 45

illness *see* disease
imbalance *see* balance
immune system 12, 103–5
  adaptogens and 129
  Ayurvedic view of 110–13
  effects of stress 141
  exercise and 126
  free radicals and 75
  and inflammation 119
  rejuvenation and 102
India, Vedic culture 153
inflammation 74, 118, 119, 131, 185
ingredients 54–7, 231–45
inner silence meditation 226–9
insulin 118
insulin-like growth factor (IGF) 118
intellect (*buddhi*) 137, 138
"intestinal dysbiosis" 63
Inuit diet 115–16
inulin 131

jaggery 240
joints, cleansing herbs 95

Kabir 225
kapha 14, 21–3
  balancing 91
  characteristics 22–3
  constitutional tendencies of the mind 139
  healthy relationship with food 150
  and immune system 110
  kapha diet 67
  kapha fast 97
  out of balance 23
  yoga for 159
karma 61, 140–1
kicharee 98
kidney beans 233
kundalini 163

ladies' fingers 234
lamb 236
Latham, Peter Mere 43
"leaky gut" syndrome 63
lecithin 117
lemon 235
lentils 233
licorice 244
life expectancy 220
life force (*prana*) 37, 38, 79, 107, 108, 184–5
lifestyles 30, 197–203
like increases like 14
lime 235
linoleic acid 61
liver: alcohol damage 78
  cleansing 86–7, 93

detoxification 76
liver spots, on skin 75
livestock industry 58
local food 62
loneliness 105, 216, 218
love 205, 207–9, 217, 218–19, 222, 223
Lovelock, James 192, 193, 194
loving-kindness 208–9
lungs, cleansing 79, 87, 88, 93
lymphatic tissue 113

magnesium 40
malnutrition 39
manas 137, 138
mangoes 235
maple syrup 240
massage 27–8
  cleansing skin 87
  cultivating compassion 207
  for rejuvenation 126
  self-massage routine 170
material world 177
meat 40, 55, 58–61, 73, 119, 120, 236
medicine: food as 41–3
  orthodox medicine 106, 109
  traditional herbal medicine (THM) 107–9, 186
  see also drugs
meditation 29, 117, 164–7
  cultivating compassion 208
  meditation practices 210–11
  the practice of inner silence 226–9
  and rejuvenation 128
  walking meditation 196
melon 235
memory 137
metabolism 76
methanol 78
Metta Sutta 208–9
milk 237
millet 232
mind: Ayurvedic concept of 137–9
  body–mind 12, 25, 86, 137
  cleansing herbs 95
  constitutional tendencies 139
  and disease 140–1
  herbs to stabilize 80
  and rejuvenation 128
  strength and stillness 164–7
  thoughts 31
minerals 40, 57, 131, 133
mint 239
moksa (self-realisation) 146, 152
molasses 240
mortality 222–3
multivitamin supplements

131, 133
mung beans 233
  kicharee 98
  mung bean soup 99
mushrooms 233
mustard seeds 239
mycotoxins 73, 80
mythology 142

nasal oiling 27
nasal washing 27
natural urges, restraining 83
nature: connecting with 195–6
  consciousness and 176
  language of 13
neem 95, 244
nervous system 12, 136
"*neti, neti*" 214
neurotoxins 80
Nirvana 214–15, 217
nonviolence (*ahimsa*) 59
"nostril only" breathing 28
nutrition *see* food
"nutritional gap" 40
nuts 55, 236

oats 232
obesity 120, 149
oil supplies, "Peak Oil" 193
oils: in diet 56
  essential oils 41, 170
  massage oils 27–8, 170
  nasal oiling 27
  the Pukka pantry 238
  vegetarian diet 64
oily fish 55
ojas (essence) 110–13
olive oil 238
olives 234
omega essential fatty acids 64, 119, 120
oneness 214–15
onions 233
opiates 148
opposites balancing opposites 14
oral hygiene 26–7
oranges 235
organic food 40, 62, 187, 188–9
orthodox medicine 106, 109

pain 142–5, 222
  meditation on 210, 211
painkillers 43, 79
palming eyes 112
papaya 235
Paracelsus 43
Pasteur, Louis 25
pathway of disease 84–5
peace 146, 228–9

peaches 235
"Peak Oil" 193
peanuts 236
pears 235
peas 234
pectin 117
peppers 234
persistent organic pollutants (POPs) 81
pesticides 40, 62, 73, 80, 119
pharmaceutical drugs *see* drugs
pheasant 236
phenotypes 24
phytonutrients 41, 57, 120
pineapple 235
pippali 122–4, 244
pitta 14, 18–20
  balancing 90–1
  characteristics 19–20
  constitutional tendencies of the mind 139
  healthy relationship with food 150
  and immune system 110
  out of balance 20
  pitta diet 66
  pitta fast 97
  yoga for 157–8
plants: chlorophyll 185
  gardening 196
  prana (life force) 184
  see also herbs
platelet-derived growth factor (PDGF) 119
plums 235
poisons: bitter taste 52
  food as 41–3
pollen, flower 190–1, 242
pollution 73, 80–1
polyphenols 53, 120
pomegranate 235
population growth 192
pork 236
poverty 220
prakriti (constitution) 11
prana (life force) 37, 38, 79, 107, 108, 184–5
pranayama (control of breath) 161
prayer 141
prebiotics 131
Prescott-Allen, Robert and Christine 221
present, awareness of 226–9
processed foods 40
prosperity 220–1
prunes 235
psychoneuroimmunology 141
psychosomatic illness 140–1

psychotherapy 216–17
psychotropic hallucinogens 148
pumpkin seeds 236
pumpkins 234
pungent taste 51

qi (vital force) 107
qualities (*gunas*) 13, 47, 182–3
quinoa 232

rajas 60, 138
rasa (taste) 46
rasayana (rejuvenation) 101
raspberries 235
recreational drugs 79, 147–8
reishi mushrooms 121, 124, 244
rejuvenation 101–33
  chlorophyll and 185
  immune system 103–5, 110–13
  rejuvenating herbs 122–5
  rejuvenation plan 131–3
  rejuvenation practices for life 126–9
  yoga and 153
relationships 205–29
  awareness of the present 226–9
  cultivating compassion 207–9
  illness as a symbol 212
  life and death 222–3
  living from the heart 213
  love 218–19
  meditation practices 210–11
  which way to Nirvana? 214–17
  with ourselves 206
  work, equality, and prosperity 220–1
relaxation 136
  exercise routines 154–5
  herbs for 168–9
  and rejuvenation 128
  Yoga Nidra 170, 171–3
religion 82, 145
resolve (*sankalpa*) 171–2
resources, limits to 192–3
"restraining your natural urges" 83
rhubarb 235
rice 232
  kicharee 98
rock salt 50
root vegetables 234
rye 232

sadness 142
safety: drugs 109
  herbal medicines 108–9

saffron 239
salt 50, 240
salty taste 50
Samkhya 145
sankalpa (resolve) 171–2
Saraswati, Swami Satyananda 170, 226
sattva 60, 138
seasonal detoxification 96
seasonal food 62
seasonal influences 83
seasonal lifestyles 197–203
seaweeds 234
seeds 55, 196, 236
selenium 120
self-esteem 213, 219
self-realization (*moksa*) 146, 152, 214–16, 217
senses: inner silence meditation 226–7
  sense withdrawal 164
  "unwholesome attachment to their objects" 83
  Yoga Nidra 171
serotonin 106, 126, 144
sesame oil 170, 238
sesame seeds 236
shatavari 80, 124, 244
Shiva Nataraja 224
"silent witness" 222
skin 75, 87, 95
sleep 126
smoking 78, 117, 118, 147
Soil Association 62
soup, mung bean 99
sour cream 237
sour taste 49
soybeans 233
Space 15
spices 56
  digestive stimulation 30
  the Pukka pantry 238–40
  vegetarian diet 64
spicy taste 51
Spirit 219
spirituality, vegetarian diet 61
spirulina 191, 242
spring routine 198–9
squash 234
statins 115–17
strawberries 236
strength and stillness 135–73
stress: Ayurvedic view of 136
  effects of 141
  heart and 114
  and immune system 105, 112
  relaxation routines 154–5
  stress hormones 126, 128
  symptoms of 136
  toxicity and 73
  yoga and 152

strokes 116
suffering 142–5, 146, 222
  meditation on 210, 211
sugar 40, 48, 57, 73, 118, 240
summer routine 199–200
sun, life force 184
sunflower oil 238
sunflower seeds 236
superfoods 57, 64, 185, 190–1, 240–2
supplements 131, 133
sustainability, herbs 186–9
sweet taste 48–9
sweeteners 57, 240
symbolism 142, 212

tamas 60, 138
tannins 53
tantra 153
tastes 46–53
tea 240
teas, herbal 57, 117, 131
temperature, taste and 47
testosterone 119
thirst 57
thoughts 31
tomatoes 234
toothpaste 27
touch 170, 219
toxins: alcohol 78
  ama 71–3
  detoxification 76–7, 82, 86, 96–7, 185
  environmental toxins 73, 80–1
  free radical damage 74–7
  pathway of disease 84–5
  pharmaceutical drugs 79
  recreational drugs 79
  smoking 78
trace elements 75
traditional herbal medicine (THM) 107–9, 186
trans fats 40, 43, 73
trigunas (forces) 60, 138
trikatu 93, 244–5
triphala 92–3, 121, 245
tulsi 125, 168, 245
turkey 236
turmeric 42, 80, 95, 117, 121, 125, 240

universal forces 138

vaccinations 104
vacha 80, 245
valerian 80
vata 14, 15–17
  balancing 90
  characteristics 16–17
  constitutional tendencies of the mind 139

healthy relationship with food 150
  and immune system 110
  out of balance 17
  vata diet 65
  vata fast 97
  yoga for 156–7
Vedic culture 153
vegetables 39–40, 54, 76, 120, 233–5
vegetarian diet 58–61, 64, 120
victory breath 162
vikriti (imbalance) 14
violence 73
viruses 104
visualization 141, 172–3
vitamins 40, 57, 64, 75–6, 131, 133
vulnerability 218–19

walking 196
washing 27
water: drinking 57, 87
  livestock industry and 58
Water (element) 13, 46, 177, 180–1, 182–3
watercress 235
watermelon 236
wealth 220–1
wheat 232
wheatgrass juice 191, 242
wholeness 12
Wilber, Ken 176, 215
Wind 13, 15
wind-relieving pose 154
winter routine 202–3
"witnessing awareness" 165
work 30, 144, 220–1
wounds 119
writing, cultivating compassion 207–8

yeast 42, 240
yoga 152–3, 215
  Dattatreya 160
  for the *doshas* 156–9
  nourishing the heart 117
  for rejuvenation 126–7
  relaxation routines 154–5
  yogis 160
Yoga Nidra 170, 171–3
yogurt 237

Zen Buddhism 215, 218
zinc 40
zucchini 233

AUTHOR'S ACKNOWLEDGMENTS

This book has flown from the wellspring of inspiration I have received from so many people, places, and teachings. I am blessed to be surrounded by them and am deeply indebted, as they help me to fulfill my potential. Especially Susie, Emerson, and Calypso, for their loving guidance that moves me to live from my heart and soul. Also my parents and family, for welcoming me into their lives and giving me the freedom to be who I am. My chosen family of friends, for their acceptance, wisdom, and support; you know who you are. My teachers have been many: Swamis Satyananda, Vedantananda, Pragyamurti, and Shankardev, for your yogic insights; Kamal Das, for showing me the heights of the Himalayas; and Angus Landman, for your spiritual guidance. I am very fortunate to have found the wisdom traditions of Ayurveda, Chinese, and herbal medicine and remain eternally grateful to the community of healers that has carried these traditions. I also thank Dr. Michael Tierra, Dr. Lesley Tierra, Annie McIntyre, Ed Berger, Nadia Brydon, Dr. Jin, Vaidyas Lad, Bendale, Lele, Venkatram, and Phadke, as well as Alan Tillotson, Todd Caldecott, Roy Upton, David Winston, David Hoffman, Donny Yance, Professor Jan Meulenbeld, Dr. Dominik Wujastyck, Alex Hankey, and Dr. Donn Brennan, for their direct and indirect inspiration. For their Indological, spiritual, and uniquely pedantic insights: Dr. James Mallinson, Dr. Alexander Watson, and Dr. Matthew Clarke. To Mike Brook, Tadesh Korbusz, Ben Heron, Benjamin Joliffe, Andrew Darnton, Vikas Bhat, Scott Cote, and Kevin Casey, who are beaming lights of herbo-ecological wisdom. To Tim Westwell and everyone at Pukka Herbs, for the fulfillment of a dream, and Nina and David Thompson for making Pukka Herbs beautiful. To everyone at Quadrille, especially Anne Furniss, Pauline Savage, and Nicola Davidson. Mr. Suresh ji, for literary insights. To Krishna Das, for his soothing bhajans. To the Cam brook, my garden, and bees. You are all continual inspirations for my head and *hridaya*. Thank you.

This book is for my patients. May your dreams come true.